See Here

By

Virginia Cantarella

Printed in Victoria, Canada

Written and illustrated by Virginia Cantarella, Member of the Association of Medical Illustrators
Design by Virginia Cantarella

National Library of Canada Cataloguing in Publication Data
Cantarella, Virginia
　　　　See here / Virginia Cantarella.
ISBN 1-55395-734-2
　　　　1. Ophthalmology--Popular works. I. Title.
RE51 C36 2003　　　　617.7　　　　C2003-900791-X

TRAFFORD

This book was published on-demand in cooperation with Trafford Publishing.
On-demand publishing is a unique process and service of making a book available for retail sale to the public taking advantage of on-demand manufacturing and Internet marketing. On-demand publishing includes promotions, retail sales, manufacturing, order fulfilment, accounting and collecting royalties on behalf of the author.

For information on ordering this book contact the publisher at:
Suite 6E, 2333 Government St., Victoria, B.C. V8T 4P4, CANADA
Phone　　250-383-6864　　　Toll-free　1-888-232-4444 (Canada & US)
Fax　　　250-383-6804　　　E-mail　　sales@trafford.com
Web site　www.trafford.com　TRAFFORD PUBLISHING IS A DIVISION OF TRAFFORD HOLDINGS LTD.
Trafford Catalogue #03-0097　　　www.trafford.com/robots/03-0097.html

10　　　9　　　8　　　7　　　6　　　5　　　4　　　3　　　2

Acknowledgements

*I*n 1970, I was a housewife with two children and little work experience. I had done some drawings for Dr. Austin Fink, my ophthalmologist, and some others for the Department of Biology at Columbia University. Richard Troutman took me on after seeing the drawings I had done for Dr. Fink. I was to illustrate the text that would change ophthalmic surgery from a primitive art to the high science that we know today. I wish to thank Dr. Troutman for never wavering in his faith in my abilities and for the hours he spent teaching me what I had to know, always with patience and encouragement. I wish to thank Eugenia Klein, whose capable editing and friendship helped me grow into the task. Thanks go to Dr. Austin Fink, who got me started, taught me about the basic anatomy of the eye, and acted as mentor and friend.

I wish to thank Catherine Duffek who suggested I get serious about writing and publishing this book, read the manuscript and had many good suggestions for making it more coherent and interesting. And my darling Sarah Shonbrun, my daughter thanks to a second marriage, who has edited the manuscript with intelligence, insight and, best of all, humor.

And last, I wish to thank Merle Gonzalez, who built the chest that housed all the artwork for that first book and the many others that followed. Without that wonderful chest I never could have organized the enormous amount of material that I had to deal with. And thanks go to his wife Charlotte, who cared for my children with humor and imagination, and kept my house running while I worked long hours on the illustrations.

Table of Contents

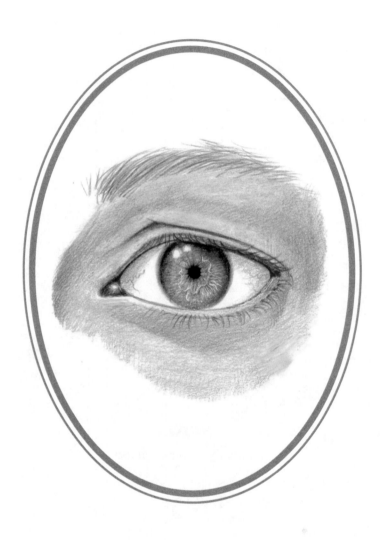

My Eye

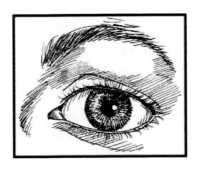

Chapter I

As I See It

*H*ow do we see? Why do we see? What is seeing? What do we see? Most of our information and knowledge comes to us through our eyes, yet most of us know very little about them.

When I was four years old and still taking naps, I would lie on my bed looking out the window. All there was to see was the sky, but I also saw little shapes like question marks or squiggles that drifted upward after my gaze was lifted or downward after my gaze was lowered. I was fascinated by them and would look in all directions to see what these little things would do. I could always entertain myself with them if sleep didn't come. I still have them, some new ones and darker ones as well. They're called floaters: debris of some sort in the vitreous humor, the gel-like fluid that fills the back of the eye. Many people have them. Some are very bothered by them, but, for the most part, they are harmless.

The eye became my world. I earned my living illustrating medical textbooks on all kinds of eye surgery. I spent much time exploring the anatomy of the eye, and the structures that surround it, to help me to understand the surgery I was asked to illustrate. My curiosity about how the eye works, how it is constructed, seemed never satisfied. Whenever I was asked to draw a new area of the eye or a new procedure, I continued my research.

It was a problem with my own eye that first got me involved with eye surgery and medical illustration. In 1963, my son, who was then an infant, hugged me and accidentally sliced my cornea with his little fingernail. I went in agony to my ophthalmologist, Dr. Austin Fink. Fink knew that I was interested in medical illustration, so while treating me he asked if I could do some drawings for him. His former illustrator had moved from New York and he wanted someone with whom he could work closely.

I had toyed with the idea of medical illustrating while in high school, but the fine arts had lured me away during college. It was the era of the abstract expressionists, after all. After I graduated from art school reality began to set in. The world was not waiting for me to present it with paintings and I was too young and raw to know what or how I wanted to paint anyway. So I began taking little jobs doing biological illustrating. Then I did a mailing to advertise my availability. My Dr. Fink had received one of these handwritten brochures.

Two weeks after my visit with the painful corneal scratch I was invited to visit Dr. Fink at his office, but this time the bandage was off. I was out of pain, I had drawing pad and pencil in hand and he had films of cataract surgery of infants to show me. I had seen surgery only once before—hand surgery—and had fainted on that occasion. This time I didn't faint but I did have to see the first film three times before I could begin to understand what I was seeing.

Dr. Fink was very patient with me. I think he could see from what I was developing on my sketch pad that I could draw well enough. When I turned in my work a week later, he suggested that I consider illustrating ophthalmology as a career. There was a lot happening in that world and it would solve the problem of my training. I could limit my work to the eye. Sounded good to me. He then gave me a three-volume anatomy text by Werner Spalteholz to begin my studies and sent me home.

My next assignment with Dr. Fink was to draw the eye of a premature infant. He was born at five months, setting a record for prematurity in that hospital. His eyes were not fully developed. There were still small blood vessels on his corneas that disappear by the time of normal birth. I was to go in and paint what his eye looked like week by week. When I first met this wee little nameless lad he looked like a baby mouse. He didn't seem human. After the sixth week, we were on good terms. Though he was blind, I felt I was gazing into his soul. He never fussed as I handled him. Maybe he liked the attention as I would cradle his head in my hand and coo to him while I worked. I learned that his family had abandoned him. The nurses at the hospital took pity on him and adopted him, going to extraordinary lengths to save his life and nurture him. I have often wondered what happened to that little boy. I do know that he never was able to see.

Years later, when I was working with a famous retinal surgeon, I learned that prematurely born infants often have retinal and back-of-the-eye problems. This surgeon was able to clear out the back chamber of the eye, getting the retina back in place so that what retina there was could pick up light and dark and maybe the vague shape of things. When I walked into his operating room my first thought was "Where is the patient?" I was used to seeing a big person lying on the operating table. These preemies are so tiny that they hardly make a crease in the sheet. But there she was, all 10 inches of her with a little white knitted cap on her head to keep in the body heat. I wasn't sure I could handle this, but the staff and the surgeon himself were so caring, and their movements so expert, I knew nothing bad would happen. I watched a miracle performed. I have watched many.

Unlike so many areas of medicine where there is little one can do to cure a patient, or the cure is worse than the disease, ophthalmology is full of successes. The patient walks in blind, or not seeing well, and some time later walks out seeing. That is the most dramatic scenario. But from the mundane experience of putting on glasses to a corneal transplant, that is essentially what is happening.

I remember coming one day to a world-famous retinal surgeon's office to get my assignment. Everyone in the office was in a great fluster as a patient had gone into cardiac arrest. It had been so long since this doctor had dealt with anything that life threatening that he had called 911, then had to take a Valium.

I would like to take you on a journey that explores the eye and its surroundings. It is a place of beauty and mystery, science and architecture, biology and optics. You will also look at some of the more common ailments and how they are treated. Part of this journey is also about how I became a medical illustrator for some of the nation's leading ophthalmologists and some of my experiences while pursuing my career.

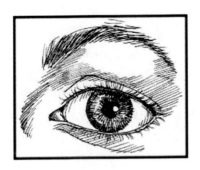

Chapter II

General Description

*I*n this book you will be looking at the globe or eyeball, the lids, the bony orbit and its contents, the lacrimal (tear) system and glands, and the sinuses. You will learn about how the eye is nourished with blood vessels and what nerves enter the orbit and what role they play in our vision. You will look at the muscles that make the eye move and those that are inside the eye to open and close the pupil to aid in focusing. You will examine the lids, and learn of the important role they play in protecting the eyes. And all of this happens in a very small area no larger than your fist.

The eye itself is only about the size of a large marble. The nature of its workings is so intricate, so exact, and so complex, it is a wonder that it evolved from such humble beginnings. The cells of simple animal life, even the outside membranes of one-celled animals, are light-sensitive.

Humans have stereoscopic vision, which means you see in three dimensions, giving you depth perception. That is only possible because both of your eyes are facing forward. For the most part animals have their eyes on the sides of their heads. Other primates (like humans) have forward-facing eyes too. Perhaps this is because they move from branch to branch high in trees or evolved from animals that did. Any bird or animal that relies on sight to catch its prey needs stereoscopic vision too. The owl is a good example.

While the eyeball is described as a globe it is not perfectly spherical, it just looks that way from the outside. The cornea, that clear tissue in front of the iris, bulges out slightly and does the primary focusing. In a healthy eye it has no blood vessels. It is full of nerve endings and is very sensitive. Behind it, really inside, behind the cornea, we see the iris and pupil. The iris is the colored part of the eye, blue, gray, hazel or brown. The pupil appears to be a black dot at the center of the iris but it is a hole—the hole we see through. Lying right behind that hole is the lens, which also aids in focusing. When the lens becomes cloudy it is called a cataract. When the lens becomes so opaque that vision is compromised, the cataract is removed. Around the cornea is the white of the eye, called the sclera. Covering the sclera is a tissue called the conjunctiva (that you hardly notice until it is bloodshot), which covers the sclera for a certain distance, then folds back, lining the inside of the lids and creating a sulcus or sac. That keeps anything from disappearing back into the orbit. That's why if you wear contact lenses, you don't worry if they get lost either up above or down below. They can't go far.

All healthy human eyes are about the same size at the same age. A newborn's eyes are about half the size of adult eyes. What makes different people's eyes look bigger or smaller is how much of the eye is covered by the lids. If you lined up a bunch of eyeballs on the table, with no lids to give them character, they'd all look pretty much the same. The apparent size of the eye is largely due to the lids, which change as the years go by. The skin, like the rest of our bodies, is subject to the pull of gravity. The skin around the eye is particularly thin and elastic. You end up with a little more than you would like. Folds and wrinkles begin to appear. Also, fat that formerly has stayed in its place gets pushed out by a slightly sagging globe, making bags under the eyes. It is not the same in everyone because characteristics are inherited and everyone's skin is different. Some may have had more exposure to the sun. There are diseases that affect the lid positions, and others that influence the position of the eye in the orbit, the bony cavity that houses the eye.

The inside of the globe is filled with aqueous and vitreous humors. The globe itself is made up of layers of tissue, starting on the inside with the retina. Behind thatt here is a pigmented layer, a vascular layer behind that, and the sclera behind that.

The lids are remarkable structures, performing all kinds of service for the protection of the eye. The lashes are part of the effort to keep things out of the eye, away from our precious corneas. The lids open and close, keeping the eye moist and preventing objects big and minuscule from getting in. When the lids blink, it is mainly the upper one closing onto the lower lid in an involuntary motion. The lower lid can rise slightly with voluntary motion. You squint with the lids to assist in seeing, in the same way that looking though a pinhole will sharpen an image. Embedded in the lids are the lacrimal glands and nestled between eye and nose is a tunnel of bone which contains the lacrimal sac. The glands produce tears and the sac draws them off into the nasal cavity, making your nose run.

With your fingertips you can feel the rim of the orbit all around your eyes. They are roughly cone-shaped, with the eyeball like the dollop of ice cream in the cones, only the cones are lying on their sides. Attached to the eyeball are the muscles that move the eye.

The sinuses are hollow areas within the bones of the skull. Without them our heads would be too heavy to hold up. There is a sinus cavity above the eyes, one below each eye, many little ones between them and behind them. They surround the orbits and, if ruptured from a blow or accident, can endanger the eye.

A Summer's Work

Dr. Richard Troutman was a good friend of my ophthalmologist, Dr. Fink. They had been colleagues for years and worked at Downstate Medical Center together. When Dr. Troutman's medical illustrator decided to quit, it left him with an important book just started and in need of someone to complete the drawings. It was my good fortune that his illustrator did not gauge the importance of that book for it helped to change the way ophthalmic surgery would be done from then on by introducing the use of the surgical microscope for eye surgery along with all the specially designed microsurgical instruments. Until then, ophthalmic surgeons wore glasses called loupes. They looked like regular glasses but had manifying devices called oculars in the middle of each lens. When the surgeon moved his head, the whole field moved. Also, the magnification was minimal.

Fink introduced me to Troutman, then showed my drawings to him. Dr. Troutman's first question was, "Can you draw eyes?" Next, before I even had a chance to answer, he asked me to join him in surgery the following Tuesday. I was to be there at 7:30 a.m. sharp. I got up at 5 a.m. and managed to show up in the correct operating room just as things were getting started. I watched the surgery through the observer's scope with Dr. Troutman explaining every step of the procedure. I didn't faint. Well, not in surgery. I almost did when, afterwards, he handed me three thousand dollars worth of instruments in a beautiful blue felt case. He told me he was ordering a student's version of the operating microscope to be delivered to me the following week. I was hired. We were going to start with the chapter on instruments. I was going away for the summer and could work with him by phone, mailing him my drawings. He would mail them back with corrections. Those were the days before faxes and e-mail. We were not just drawing what these instruments looked like but how they worked and the mechanical principles behind the way they were designed. I went off for the summer with my new microscope and all my instruments.

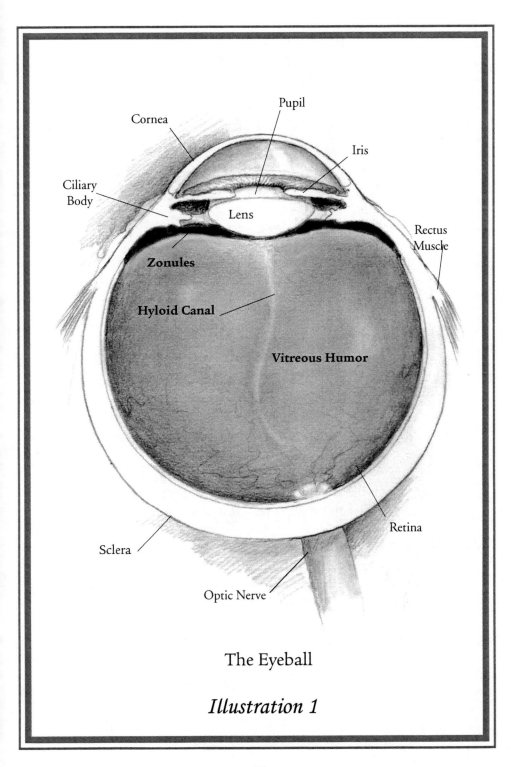

Cornea

Pupil

Iris

Ciliary Body

Lens

Rectus Muscle

Zonules

Hyloid Canal

Vitreous Humor

Retina

Sclera

Optic Nerve

The Eyeball

Illustration 1

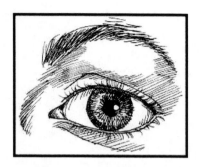

Chapter III

The Eyeball

MEASUREMENTS

*I*n the world of medicine small things are measured in terms of millimeters—abbreviation mm. One mm is about one thirty-second of an inch

An eyeball with the cornea facing you would appear round. If you looked at an eyeball with the cornea above—at the north pole, so to speak—you would note the bulge of the cornea. The cornea and the globe are two incomplete spheres. The cornea, if made to complete its sphere, would be the smaller sphere; the sclera would be the larger one. [Illustration 1.] The curvature of the cornea is a more perfect sphere. The sclera is slightly wider at the equator, but, because of the bulge of the cornea, the diameter measured from north to south is 24 mm, whereas the diameter measured across the equator is about 23.5 mm or about fifteen-sixteenths of an inch. The diameter of the cornea at the point where it intersects the sclera is about 12 mm—a little less than a half an inch.

The eye sits in the front part of the orbit. It is slightly closer to the roof of the orbit than the floor and slightly closer to the outside than the nasal side.

The eye is divided into two segments or chambers—the anterior chamber and the posterior chamber. [Illustration 2.]

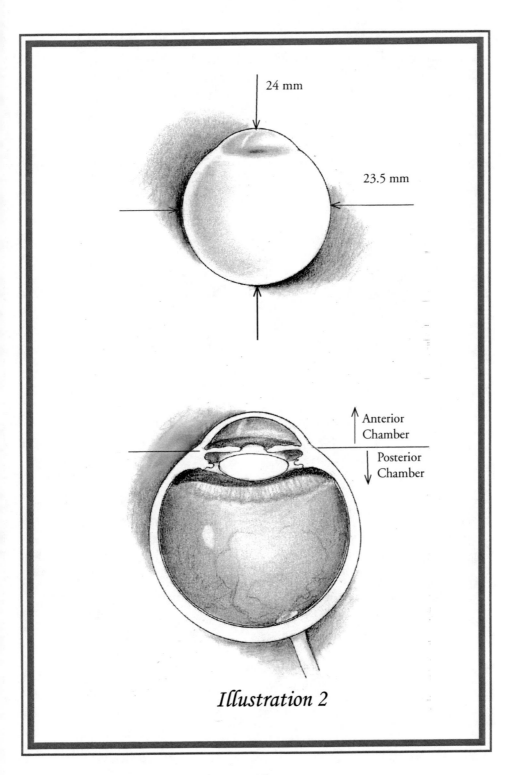

24 mm

23.5 mm

Anterior
Chamber

Posterior
Chamber

Illustration 2

Everything from the iris forward is called the anterior chamber. It includes the iris; the angle, where the iris meets the cornea; the aqueous humor, the fluid in the front of the eye; and the cornea. The posterior chamber includes the lens, the zonules, the ciliary body, the vitreous humor, and the retina. These and related structures will be described and explained.

CAMEL CACA

Not only did Dr. Troutman hire me to do the drawings for his book on Microsurgery of the Eye, he also wanted me to design the cover. In fact, he planned on doing three books and he wanted all three covers to be related. I traveled St. Louis to visit the publisher, C.V. Mosby, and our editor, Eugenia Klein. I learned how covers were made and then was given a batch of swatches of the colors and materials of which they were made. There were hundreds of them. I chose a different color for each of the three books. The first book would be a beige-khaki color, the second rust, and the third a blue-green. I drew a graphic representation of the iris behind a cornea, done in black embossed in the material, and the lettering was to be copper, with some of that copper showing in the graphic as well. The fonts for the lettering were chosen and it all came together. The design people at Mosby were pleased and I thought it would make a good-looking cover that could be modified for the future two books.

They made up a dummy cover to send to Dr. Troutman along with color samples for the other two. When I saw him in the operating room that next Tuesday morning he seemed very pleased with what I had done. That evening, however, he phoned. I could hear his wife in the background saying, "The color of this book looks like camel caca." I pretended I hadn't heard. When he expressed concern about the color I think I said something like, "Trust me, it will be fine." He did. There were no more questions about it.

At the following Academy of Ophthalmology, the book was

18

presented by Mosby. Dr. Troutman told me afterwards that his colleagues who also had written books were curious about the cover. Not only did they like it, they wanted to know how they could have something similar rather than the standard medical textbook cover. Years later, when the other two books were published, Mosby used my original idea and design. They made a handsome and original three volume set. When I got to know Dr. Troutman's wife better in later years we laughed about the camel caca. By then Dr. Troutman's books were so sought after that medical libraries couldn't keep them; they have all been stolen!

THE ANTERIOR CHAMBER

It is difficult to see the interior of the anterior chamber, particularly the angle where the iris meets and joins the sclera at the corneal-scleral junction. There is an instrument called the gonioscope which does allow a view into the angle of the anterior chamber, but it is awkward to use and the view is limited. Looking up from the iris, you see the interior of the dome of the cornea with its basement membrane of endothelial cells. Looking toward the horizon—the angle of the eye—you see several rings. The topmost, narrow and whitish, is called Schwalbe's Ring. Next, darker and broader, is the trabecular meshwork which covers Schlemm's Canal—discussed below. Beneath is a lighter and narrower ring called the scleral spur. It is the point where sclera and cornea meet. Below that are the iris processes, whitish or yellowish bands that run up to Schwalbe's Ring from the area of the root or outermost part of the iris. [See Illustration 3.]

The anterior chamber is filled with aqueous humor, a watery fluid something like lymph, that is continuously being manufactured in the ciliary body just behind the iris. Since aqueous humor is always being added to the interior of the eye, it must drain off in some way or the pressure in the eye would become too high, causing the condition known as glaucoma. The aqueous humor fills all available space in the eye, finding its way over the lens and through the pupil into the anterior chamber. In the angle of the eye, the area where the cornea meets that part of

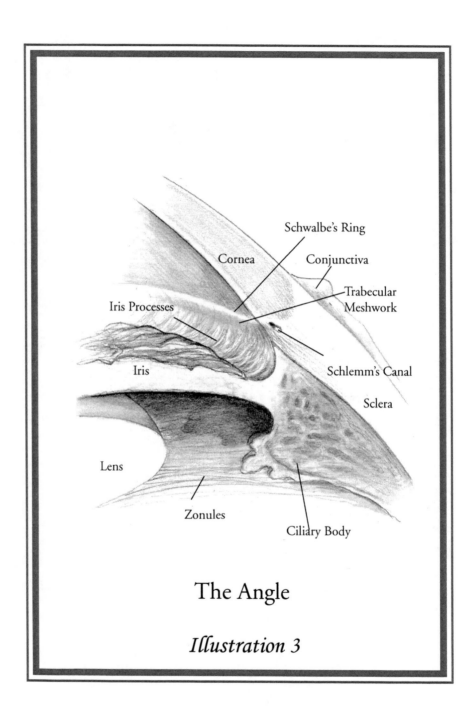

The Angle

Illustration 3

the sclera where the iris is attached, there is a channel in the sclera called Schlemm's Canal. The channel encircles the globe, sometimes as a single channel, sometimes as a double one. Its connection with the interior of the chamber is a structure called the trabecular meshwork. The mounting pressure of the aqueous humor forces it through the trabecular meshwork into the canal. From there, the aqueous is drained off into nearby veins. (The exact mechanism of how the aqueous humor reaches Schlemm's Canal was of particular interest to Dr. Fink, who wrote a paper on this research and had me illustrate it.) In a healthy eye, the amount that is drained off equals the amount that is produced, maintaining a steady pressure in the eye. That pressure maintains the shape of the eye, not allowing it to collapse. That is a concern in surgery and steps are taken, once the globe has been entered, to keep it from collapsing.

Glaucoma is caused by some kind of obstruction in the angle of the eye, keeping the aqueous humor from exiting. In open angle glaucoma the obstruction is not so apparent. Somewhere between the trabecular meshwork and Schemm's Canal, the aqueous humor is blocked from draining out of the eye. In closed angle glaucoma one can see the problem. The iris may stick to the cornea, closing off the angle, or it just might be pushed up against the cornea, creating the same problem. Closed angle glaucoma can be handled with surgery. Open angle glaucoma is treated first with drugs and then surgery if the drugs stop working. What is called a filtering bleb is created, which is a hole in the cornea that the surgeon covers with the conjunctiva so that you don't notice it so much, but the aqueous can filter out through it. In glaucoma the problem starts in the angle with the obstruction that blocks the exiting of the aqueous. The damage caused by the raised pressure in the eye is at the place in the back of the eye where the optic nerve enters along with the vessels. The raised pressure on the nerve, which is made up of all the neurons leading from the sight cells—the rods and the cones—eventually damages it, creating areas of blindness that, if unchecked, can lead to total blindness.

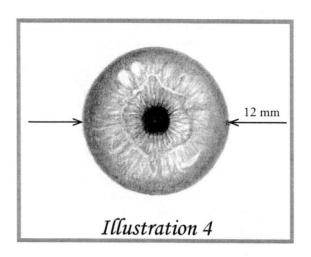

12 mm

Illustration 4

THE CORNEA

The cornea is the window of the eye. It is a clear, layered tissue and is remarkably tough. The cornea is not the same thickness all the way across. In the center, called the pupillary area, it is only about .5 mm thick and not quite twice that at its periphery. Ideally, the curvature of the cornea is a section of a sphere with a diameter of about 12 mm. [Illustration 4.] If the curvatures are not the same in all directions you have a condition called astigmatism. The cornea is the principal focusing structure of the eye, in a process called refraction. The lens only fine-tunes focusing, particularly for up-close vision. If the curvatures of the cornea are all the same, the lines of focusing will meet at a point right on the retina. If the corneal surface is uneven, or if the curve is steeper in one meridian and shallower in the other, (imaginary horizontal and vertical lines that bisect the cornea), then the lines of focusing will not meet and vision will be blurred. To visualize the steeper and flatter, or shallower, meridians, think of a football vs. a soccer ball shape. That is an exaggeration compared to the meridians of the cornea, but gives a clear idea. [Illustration 5.]

Sometimes the bisecting meridians of the cornea are of the same curvature, but are too flat, causing the lines of focusing to merge behind the cornea, producing farsightedness or presbyopia—a

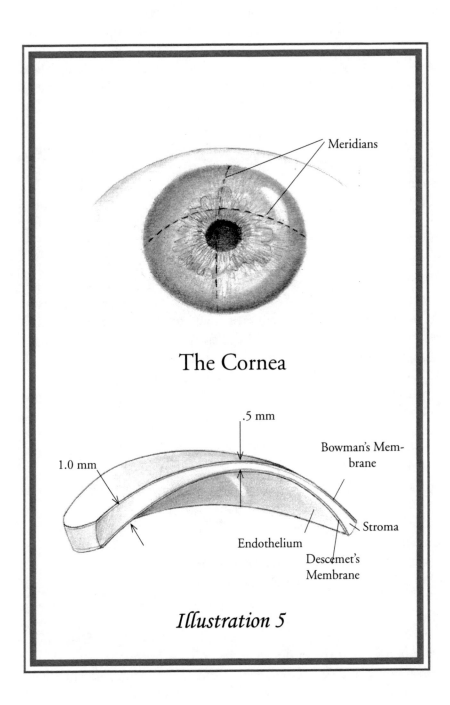

Meridians

The Cornea

.5 mm

1.0 mm

Bowman's Membrane

Stroma

Endothelium

Descemet's Membrane

Illustration 5

condition in which objects at a distance are seen clearly but those close by are out of focus. Or the corneal curves are too steep, causing the lines of focusing to merge in front of the retina, producing near- sightedness or myopia—a condition in which objects up close are in focus but those far away are not. An extra-large globe or an extra-small one can cause the same problems.

The healthy cornea has no blood vessels. They would interfere with vision. Therefore, a cut cornea heals fairly slowly, not having the kind of nourishment that tissues with blood vessels have. Nourishment to the cornea comes from the lymphatic system along with blood vessels that come right up to the edge of the cornea. Lymph bathes the cornea, seeping into it via the layers described below. It does have a nerve supply, but the nerves are so small that they are not visible without special illumination and magnification.

There are five layers, or lamina, of the cornea. The outermost is called the epithelium. It is only about five or six cells in thickness and, if scraped off the eye, will grow back or regenerate. The next layer, parallel to the curvature of the epithelium, is called Bowman's membrane. It will not regenerate, but it is much tougher than the epithelium, so is much harder to destroy, and acts as a protective layer. It is a thinner layer even than the epithelium, but is not composed of cells, rather of very fine collagen fibers that travel in all directions parallel to the surface. The body of the cornea is called the stroma. It too is made up of collagen fibers. In a living cornea, it is almost impossible to see any structure in the stromal layer and therefore it appears perfectly clear. On the inner side of the cornea are two more layers, Descemet's membrane and the endothelium. Descemet's membrane is a very tough thin layer and quite distinct from the stroma. Descemet's membrane resists infection and acts as a barrier to germs and other invaders from the outside, protecting the inner chamber. The endothelium is a layer of tissue only one cell in thickness. It is the innermost layer and the most delicate. Once endothelial cells are touched and removed, they will not regenerate. When corneal grafting is being done, the donor corneal tissue must be handled so that the endothelial layer is never touched and therefore not compromised. The layers of the cornea are called lamellae. A layer or layers of the cornea can be peeled away safely. This is helpful in conditions where the pathology (illness) does not compromise the entire depth of the cornea.[Illustration 5.]

Corneal Graft Part 1

The first time I walked into the operating theater for micro-surgery of the eye I was impressed with the quiet efficiency of everyone there. Suspended from the ceiling on a track was the operating microscope, with all its attachments. It had lights and a built-in camera. There were three microscopes; one for the surgeon, and two for observers on each side. Directly under the scope was the operating table. The patient was on the table draped for surgery with just the eye that was to be operated on exposed to view. At the head of the table was a special chair on wheels with a back support and arm rests. Dr. Troutman was seated there adjusting the microscope so that it was exactly the correct distance from the patient and in a comfortable position for him to peer into the eyepiece (oculars). At his feet was a panel of foot pedals that were used for the fine tuning of the micro-scope. One pedal raised the scope, another lowered it, and another controlled magnification or zoom, which went from roughly three-to 12-times magnification. Beside the operating table were several instrument tables made of bent stainless steel tubing, upon which rested trays arrayed with all the instruments that would be used for this particular surgery, a corneal transplant. Against the wall were cabinets with glass doors filled with boxes of instruments and other equipment that might be needed for more extensive surgeries. There was also a work table where the surgeon would prepare the graft. There was a huge wastebasket lined with plastic. Stools were placed at the position of the observer scopes and I took my place at the one to the left of the surgeon. Everyone was dressed in grayish-blue-green pajamas, some with coats, and all with paper coverings on their feet, flowered caps for the women's heads and blue-green caps for the men. And masks of course. All you could see of our faces were our eyes. There was a nurse to hand over instruments to the surgeon, gowned, gloved and masked. Another was there to get additional instruments if needed. The anesthetist, with all his equipment, sat across from me. The heart monitor made a monotonous beep beep beep. A screen showed what that beeping was about. The anesthetist kept squeezing a black rubber balloon that assisted the patient in breathing while he was under anesthesia.

Everyone knew their responsibilities and where to be at any given moment. Except me. Suddenly the instrument nurse said in what sounded to me like a chilly tone, "Doctor, your medical illustrator has touched your sleeve, contaminating you." The doctor replied, "It will take two weeks for those little buggies to travel from my elbow to my fingers. I think we're all right here." Everyone laughed, including the nurse, and surgery began.

THE IRIS

The iris is the colored part of the eye. It is like a disc with a hole in the middle called the pupil. The pupil becomes larger or smaller depending on how bright the light is. The brighter the light, the smaller the pupil. It works like a camera's lens. The opening or aperture in front of the lens broadens to allow more light in if there isn't very much light, and it becomes smaller to keep too much light from entering if it is very bright. The pupil also becomes smaller to aid in focusing. If you are nearsighted or farsighted you can look though a small pinhole in a piece of paper and you will find that you can see clearly. Nearsighted or farsighted, it will help you focus. (This is good information if you're ever stuck in a phone booth without your glasses and need to look up a number.) The opening and closing of the pupil is controlled by muscle fibers in the iris.

The body of the iris is soft, like undulating velvet, with pockets called crypts, and folds, and furrows. The body, or stroma, is made up of collagen fibers in which are found pigment cells, blood vessels and nerves, and the muscles that close the pupil. Overlying them, reaching all the way back to the root, are the dilator muscles that open the pupil. The root of the iris is the part that is attached to the inner wall of the sclera and the ciliary body beneath it. The bottom layer of the iris is called the pigment epithelium. It is a brown pigmented layer.

When babies are born there is very little pigment in the stroma of their irises and as they grow, pigment cells form, giving the true color to the child's eye. That is the reason that the color of the eye changes from baby blue to brown or hazel, or remains blue if little pigment is formed. The reason a baby's eyes look blue is that one sees the pigment layer through the stroma of the iris and it appears blue even though that pigment layer is dark brown. It is the same principle that makes mountains look blue in the distance because of the atmosphere in between. Babies born with brown eyes are born with a full complement of brown pigment in the stromas of their irises.

CORNEAL GRAFT PART 2

There was some tension in the room. The eye bank was still testing the newly arrived corneas to be sure the donor material was good. If not, the surgery would have to be postponed until good donor material arrived at the eye bank. Patients must be scheduled for surgery, but in earlier days of corneal grafting donor material was only good for about one day. There would be a mad dash to the hospital where a person who had donated their corneas had died. Usually a Fellow or intern would make the run, bringing the fresh eyes back to the eye bank, which was located on the top floor of the hospital. There the technicians would examine the corneas under a particular kind of microscope called a slit lamp to be sure they were good before sending one of them down to the operating room. The slit lamp projects a strip of light that can be moved over the surface of the cornea, allowing the technician to spot any irregularities.

FACING MY DREAD

I remember thinking: I can handle surgery but I'm not sure I want to see an eye removed from a cadaver. Two days later Dr. Troutman called to tell me that the next chapter we were going to work on concerned preparation of the donor eye. I would have to watch and draw pictures of an enucleation—the removal of an eye from a cadaver. I was to be on call and was given a yellow emergency card that I could place in my car window so I wouldn't have to worry about parking at the hospital. I dreaded that call but it came soon enough. As I drove out on the Brooklyn-Queens Expressway I kept thinking of excuses I could make to avoid this experience. When I reached the hospital the admitting officer asked for my permit. I had no permit. I looked to the Fellow who was going to do the enucleation. He had no permit for me either. I insisted they call Manhattan Eye and Ear Hospital and ask for Dr. Troutman. I was sure this matter would be cleared up directly. They called and it was and suddenly I could have kicked myself because here I was, cleared to see what I had been dreading. The Fellow, however, was an empathetic chap. I think he could read every thought in my head. He undoubtedly had felt the same way his first time out. As we went down the stairs to the morgue he asked me if I was having some collywobbles. I nodded yes. He told me not to worry. With eye number one he would have me serve as his nurse, handing over instruments, so I could get used to it. It turned out he was a funny man. As he worked away, he got me laughing, and pretty soon it was all right. With the second eye I took my notes and sketched with ease. The series I did for the book were some of the nicest drawings I had done.

Even though it is just the corneas that are used, the whole eye must be removed from the cadaver. The missing eyes are replaced by round balls that look something like ping-pong balls so that the face will still look normal for any viewing. Once at the eye bank, the corneas, with a collar of sclera, are cut away and placed in a little jar with preserving fluid. In the 1970's they had to be used within about 12 hours. Today they can be kept safely for 48 hours, taking some of the drama and tension out of the situation.

Corneal Graft Part 3

As surgery began, the lights were lowered and a spotlight was focused on the patient. Dr. Troutman made the final adjustments in the positioning of the microscope. The lids were held open with a lid speculum, a small wire device that works like a spring, catching the lids and keeping them open and out of the field of the operation. An assistant dripped saline solution over the cornea to keep it moist. Troutman asked for the superior rectus fixation forceps. This forceps is used to pick up the superior rectus muscle, the muscle at the top of the eye, so that a fixation suture can be passed beneath it and then attached to the towel wrapped around the head of the patient. This held the globe still, with the cornea directly beneath the microscope and good visibility for the surgeon. Next, a fixation ring was sewed onto the sclera encircling the cornea. This ring helped to maintain the shape of the globe and gave the surgeon something on which to stabilize his instruments as the donor tissue was being sutured into the recipient wound edge.

THE LIMBUS

The limbus is the area where the cornea and sclera join. It is a slightly fuzzy or grayish ring at the edge of the cornea. A lip of sclera projects over the edge of the iris. That greyish ring is the outside edge of the iris as seen through that very thin projection of sclera. [Illustration 12.]

THE DISASTER

Dr. Troutman's success-rate statistices were some of the best in the country, in spite of the fact that his patients were mostly referrals from other doctors when a case was difficult or in trouble. For all the years I observed surgery I only saw one procedure where things went wrong. This was a surgery being monitored by Dr. Troutman. The surgeon was a Fellow doing a case from the clinic. The man had been shot in the eye with a BB gun. They believed the pellet was still in the eye. An X-ray and a sonogram did not show where it was. The Fellow made his incision close to the entry wound, which was located in the sclera just beyond the limbus. He could not find the pellet. By assuming that the pellet had traveled to the other side of the globe, he created more damage with the probe, searching for it there. It turned out that it was right next to the entry wound and if it had been noticed in the beginning, no further damage would have been done to the eye.

I was interested to see how Troutman was going to handle this disaster. First, he took responsibility himself for the problem, explaining to the patient exactly what had happened. He also took an encouraging attitude toward the Fellow, without belittling the seriousness of the mistake. He acknowledged that the Fellow's assumptions had been reasonable. In the future, however, it would be wise to start looking for a foreign object near the entry wound first. He then presented the case to all the other Fellows and interns so they could learn from the experience.

THE POSTERIOR CHAMBER

If the posterior chamber were cut in half at its equator and you could look into each interior, they would look something like Illustrations 6 and 7. Taking the part near the lens, we see the lens in the middle, attached at its outer rim by many little filaments called zonules that radiate out to the ciliary body. The ciliary body is a structure that grows out beneath the iris with many projecting fingers from which the zonules originate. The diameter of the lens is about 9 or 10 mm. From below, the ciliary body looks like about 72 wiggly bodies radiating out, as all we can see of it are the processes, each about 1 mm in length. About 1.5 mm farther out we see a toothed ring called the ora serrata. The ciliary process smooths out as it goes towards the ora serrata and that part is called the pars plana (plain fields). The ora serrata marks the beginning of the retina.

Now, looking at the other hemisphere, we see the retina and the point where it radiates out from the optic nerve. The inner base of this sphere is called the fundus. There are two "centers," one more obvious than the other. The more obvious one is where veins and arteries enter the back of the eye and begin spreading out in two major and two minor arching branchings to cover almost the entire retinal surface. The arteries are narrower than the veins and redder, the veins are bluish. The arteries carry fresh blood saturated with oxygen and nutrients from the lungs to the cells and structures they are designated to nourish. Veins are filled with the blood that is carrying off the waste products and carbon dioxide from those cells. When a light is shone on the back of the eye, the arteries are distinguished by a very evident white highlight, whereas the veins are duller. The veins and arteries run roughly in the same directions but do not stay parallel or close so as not to cast a shadow on the retina, interfering with vision. The artery emerges nasal to the vein; that is, on the side nearest the nose. They emerge out of what is called the optic disc, a whitish and almost round disc that has a pale orangy-pink border. The disc is on the same plane as the retina but it is the retina's weak point because the sclera and other layers are penetrated by the optic nerve and vessels. To strengthen it, the disc is made up of many little striations forming what is called the cribiform plate, which is the whiter part of the disc. There is no retinal layer over the disc and it is the "blind

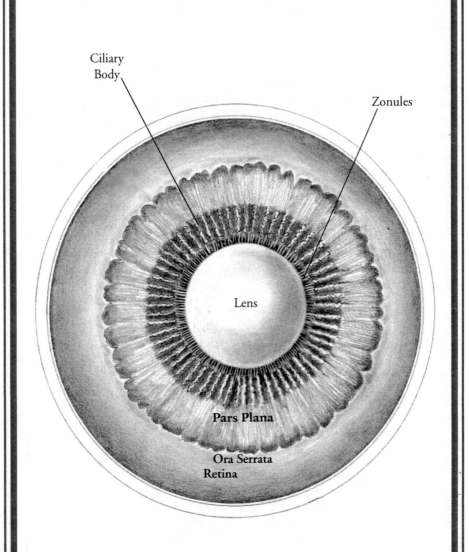

Ciliary Body

Zonules

Lens

Pars Plana

Ora Serrata
Retina

Interior of the Eye Looking Toward the Lens

Illustration 6

cribiform plate caused by raised pressure in the eye that damages the optic nerve in glaucoma.

The other center is subtle. Veins and arteries seem to swing around, above and below, like graceful branches, and then stop, leaving an oval and empty area with no vessels. This area is called the macula. The area is slightly darker red than the rest of the retina. At its center is a slight indentation called the foveola, surrounded by the fovea. The retina is thinner in the fovea and has only cones. Rods and cones are the two different kinds of receptor cells that distinguish light and dark, and color. There is no visible demarcation of these areas, but I have drawn circles in the illustration to show where these areas are. The macula is the area of central vision, that which is right in front of us. We have all heard of the dread disease, usually of older age, called macular degeneration in which central vision is compromised. Thanks to laser surgery its progress can be slowed down considerably. Peripheral vision is that which is outside of the central vision. The farther out you go on the retina, the more peripheral the vision becomes. [Illustration 7.]

THE GRASSHOPPER MIND

I worked for Dr. Francis L'Esperance, the famous retinal surgeon who developed the use of the laser in retinal surgery. Dr. L'Esperance was a brilliant man whose mind worked like a grass-hopper. You never knew where it was going to land. But that is ahead of my story. When I was called for my first interview with him, I was recently divorced and poor as a church mouse, wearing hand-me-down clothes from my cousin's wife who had recently died. When I put on that old gray coat, I noticed that the lining of the sleeves was coming out. I stuffed them back up, but felt all wrong. L'Eesperance's office was at 71st Street. and 5th Avenue. For those that don't know New York City, that is a posh neighborhood. I took the subway to 68th Street. When I got out I saw a shop with women's coats and boots. There was a SALE sign on the window. I went in and with the last money I had in the bank bought a beautiful wool coat and high boots that zipped up the back. Smashing. I threw away my old coat, stuffed my shoes in my bag, and went to my meeting with Dr. L'Esperance. I got the job.

The Nasal Side

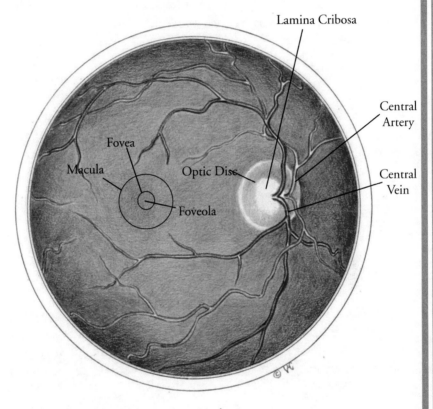

Lamina Cribosa

Central
Artery

Central
Vein

Fovea

Macula

Optic Disc

Foveola

The Temporal Side

The Fundus

Illustration 7

I was to illustrate L'Esperance's book on Diabetic Retinopathy. My next meeting with him was on an early July day and he suggested we meet in Central Park. It was beautiful out and there would be no distractions from the office. We sat on a bench overlooking a pond. There were children sailing their boats, and others throwing little firecrackers at the boats. Dr. L'Esperance was entranced and soon was throwing fire crackers along with the ten-year-olds. We didn't get much done. For the next meeting he suggested I come to his home in Englewood, New Jersey. He had a beautiful place and we worked out in the back porch overlooking his gracious lawn and gardens. We worked well for two hours, then his wife called us for lunch. On the table, beside soup and dainty sandwiches, was a huge bottle of wine. When I got home that evening I looked at my notes. The morning's notes were clear as crystal. The afternoon's were not translatable.

Our next meeting was on a train to Baltimore. He had invited me to attend a meeting on laser surgery of the retina. The idea was that we would work on the train ride down and back. Good idea, except that the train bed was not smooth. My notes, again, were hardly legible. Fortunately the meeting was very informative for me so the trip was not an entire loss.

It is somewhat of a mystery to me how I ever was able to get the information for his book. Each visit was erratic for one reason or another, but we did get it finished and the book came together, with the indispensable help of our editor, Eugenia Klein.

The laser is a mechanism that focuses and concentrates light on one spot, producing a burn. This burn, called cauterization, can arrest the disease process in several ways. It can tack down a detached retina, stop the bleeding of a small hemorrhage, or slow down the development of macular degeneration. In diabetic retinopathy, the little blood vessels in the back of the eye can proliferate, multiplying in number, branches and dimension, blocking the retina and obscuring sight. The laser burns them away and the cauterization keeps them from bleeding.

Before surgery could begin on the recipient eye, the donor tissue, called the donor button, had to be prepared. This was done at some distance from the patient on a small work table. The cornea, still with its collar of scleral tissue, was brought to the operating room in a small jar. It was removed with a forceps—using care to grasp the scleral collar to avoid disrupting the endothelial tissue on the underside of the cornea—and laid in a petri dish with the epithelial side down. In the 70's, the corneal graft and the recipient corneas were cut by hand using a trephine. A trephine is a round knife that looks like a tube about 8 mm in diameter. After examining the trephine blade, Dr. Troutman centered it over the donor cornea, then pressed down, cutting the donor "button." The top of the button was marked so that it would go into the recipient with the same orientation that it had in the original eye. The donor button was then transported in a petri dish to the area of the surgery.

Now Troutman was ready to cut the recipient cornea, the cornea of the patient, with a trephine of the same size. This was a little trickier, as there was nothing solid behind it. Once the cornea was entered, the pressure of the eye could drop and the ring sewed to the sclera would maintain the shape of the globe. After the trephine was gently placed in the center of the cornea, it was twisted slowly while gently pressing down until there was an escape of aqueous humor, the sign that the cornea had been penetrated in at least one spot. Troutman removed the trephine and finished cutting the recipient cornea with a pair of scissors

Trephine

that had blades curved to exactly match the curve of the opening being made. There were both left- and right-cutting scissors. This was necessary, as you can't move the head of the patient for easier access the way you can move the donor button. The patient's defective cornea was then taken to the laboratory for pathological examination.

Today there is much more sophisticated instrumentation for cutting both the recipient and donor corneas, some of it developed by D. Troutman.

THE CILIARY BODY

When the white of the eye is dissected away, what is left looks a little like a grape on a stem—the stem being the optic nerve. Uva is Latin for grape. The ciliary body is part of the uveal tract which begins in the posterior chamber as the choroid—the vascular (containing blood vessels) layer of the posterior chamber lying just behind the retina—continuing to the ciliary body and then ending in the interior of the iris. The ciliary body contains the ciliary muscles. At the ends of the ciliary processes, which extend from the body, are the filaments called zonules that attach to the lens. [Illustration 6.] The zonules are tightened or loosened by the action of the ciliary muscles. When the zonules release, the curvature of the lens becomes more convex, allowing for more close-up vision. This is called accommodation. The situation begins to change at around the age of 40. You begin to find you need to hold the newspaper farther and farther away from your eyes to be able to read. As you age, the lens hardens and it is more difficult for the zonules to change the lens' shape. Finally the time comes to get reading glasses or bi- or tri-focals. One famous corneal surgeon I know got his glasses from the rack at his local drugstore. They do the job just fine if you have no other problems such as astigmatism or near-sightedness.

The ciliary processes are not pigmented and when seen from below appear as light wiggly-looking ridges surrounded by darker-pigmented valleys, forming a circle around the lens. [Illustration 6.] These processes are filled with blood vessels; mainly veins. This is the most vascularized portion of the eye. During surgery it is important that the uveal tract be treated with the greatest care to avoid bleeding within the eye.

CORNEAL GRAFT PART 5

Before the graft was placed in the eye, a small hole was cut in the iris to allow the aqueous humor free access to the front of the eye, just in case the lens adhered to the iris. Called an iridectomy, it was done at the very top of the iris where it would not be noticed once the surgery was over. Dr. Troutman then picked up the donor button with a tiny spatula from the Teflon™ block, where it had been kept since being cut, and transferred it to the surgical field. Because the donor cornea had been kept moist, it adhered to the spatula, so that when the spatula was turned over to place the donor tissue in the recipient opening it didn't slip or fall out. Because the top of the button had been marked, it was placed in its new eye with the same orientation it had in its original eye.

LAYERS OF THE BACK OF THE EYE

The retina is the first layer on the inside of the back of the globe. That is the layer with the rods and cones: the nerve cells that pick up what we see. Both are photoreceptor (light sensing) cells, each of which has a fine hair-like extension called a neuron that runs to and becomes one of the many strands making up the optic nerve. It then continues to the optic chiasma where the two optic nerves cross and merge. Each then continues to the area of the brain that translates the nerve impulses into the images that we see. You could think of it as the electrical lines that connect every light and appliance in a home to the line at the pole on a street, where it joins a larger line, that eventually reaches the main generator where the electricity is produced. There has to be a continuous connection from beginning to end or the light or appliance won't work. Rods and cones are long and narrow cells that look very much alike. The cone cells are sensitive to color and to spatial differences. They need good light to do their job. The rod cells are sensitive to light and dark, the "chiaroscuro" of things, and are better adapted to night or dim-light vision. The image that is focused on the retina is upside down. It is the brain that turns it around so we see the world right-side-up.

Embedded in the retina are the retinal vessels. The retinal artery arrives at the interior of the globe by traveling alongside the optic nerve, entering it near the globe. It enters the chamber from the middle of the optic nerve, very close to the vein, which has traveled up the interior of the optic nerve to make its entrance. From there, the veins and arteries spread out, making a large arc on the temporal side and a smaller one on the nasal side. This is one area of the body where physicians can observe veins and arteries. They can even detect a slight pulsation, in the arteries especially. The veins and arteries branch and rebranch until they are very fine capillaries, which nourish and cleanse the retina. If a small artery is blocked, the area that it nourishes becomes a blind spot on the retina.

The retina is extremely fragile. It's soft and easily torn. When I was dissecting eyes, I found it impossible to remove a retina and keep it as a whole structure. It disintegrated when I grasped it with anything. A retinal detachment means that the retina has separated from the underlying tissue, allowing fluid to seep in behind it. Vision gets distorted, or, if the retina tears, is even more impaired.

The next layer, lying right behind the retina, is called the pigment epithelium. It is the pigmented layer that continues all the way to the underside of the iris. It plays a dual role in lining the retina, helping to maintain the rod and cone cells and working as an antireflective mechanism keeping light from bouncing back onto the rods and cones to distort the images. In the historical development of the eye from the most primitive form, you find dark pigment cells surrounding or backing the photosensitive cells for exactly the same purpose.

The layer backing the pigment epithelium is called the choroid. It is almost entirely made up of blood vessels. The vessels are arranged in three layers, with the largest on the scleral side and the smallest, capillary-sized, on the retinal side. The arterial vessels bring nourishment to the retina. The vessels together help maintain temperature and pressure in the eye. The veins form a kind of whorl shape exiting via four large veins, each called a vena verticosa, which protrude through the sclera. The ciliary arteries enter in the front of the eye near the muscle attachments and in the rear next to the optic nerve.

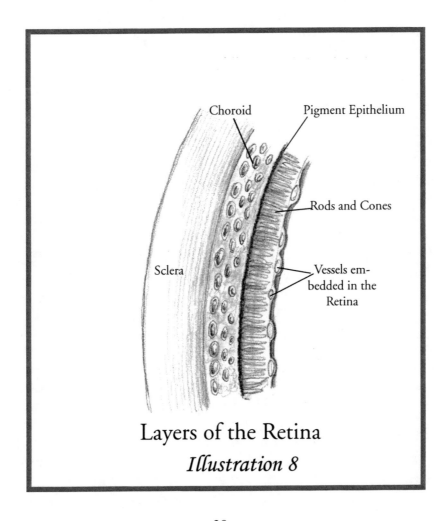

Layers of the Retina
Illustration 8

To differentiate between the two kinds of vessels: there are the vessels that enter the eye with the optic nerve and are embedded in the retinal layer; these nourish only the retina. Then there are the vessels in the choroid, which enter through the sclera at the different points discussed above. These also nourish the retina as well as the optic nerve, the pars plana, the ciliary body, the iris, all the way to the conjunctiva and other parts of the anterior chamber.

The final layer is the sclera, the white of the eye. It gets thicker—from about .6 mm at the sides to about 1 mm at the rear. The sclera is made up of collagen fibers that run in all directions, but parallel to the surface of the sclera. These are tough, non-elastic fibers that provide a sturdy base into which the muscles that move the eye are inserted. This toughness also provides a good protection for the delicate structures inside the eye.

Corneal Graft Part 6

The most dramatic and the most boring part of the surgery was the suturing of the donor button to the recipient opening. The needles were curved, like upholstery needles, only about the size of a baby's fingernail clipping. The suture was swaged—that is, directly joined to the end of the needle and not going through a little eye—so there was no lump at the joining of the filament to the needle. The filament looked as if it were growing right out of the end of the needle. The suture, or thread, was a monofilament made of synthetic material that was so fine it could only be seen under the microscope. It could get lost if not handled very carefully. The attending nurse was trained in the exact procedure for handing it to the surgeon, presenting it on the back of a gloved hand so that it could easily be grasped with the needle holder. The surgeon could then bring it directly under the microscope where the thread was clearly seen. The needles were much too tiny to be handled with fingers and were always handled with needle holders. The needle holders for microsurgery had very delicate pointed graspers that held the needle and guided it through the tissue.

In the early days of grafting, before the microscope was used, the graft was sewn with silk sutures. Under the microscope the thread looked like rope when compared with the slender and smooth modern sutures. The needles had "eyes" as well.

Some sutures come "double-armed," some are "single-armed," which means there is either a needle at both ends of the suture or only at one end. For grafting, the surgeon needed a single-armed suture. An interrupted suture is one in which the surgeon takes one bight (or stitch), attaching one tissue to the other, then ties a knot. A running suture is one in which the surgeon takes one stitch after another, either completing the circle, in the case of a graft, or completing a line, in which case the suture is fixed with a special knot at each end to keep it in place.

Tying knots was also a very important aspect of surgery. Sailors would understand. Right over left, left over right was the way to go—the old fashioned square knot. In this surgery, however, sometimes three "throws" would be made. A slip knot would do just that—slip— especially with suture material that was so smooth.

Tying the knot

So that young doctors could learn from our book I had to show what the knots looked like. Because the suture material was so fine, even with my microscope I could see the knots only as black dots. It was a real problem until the day I had to go to my butcher to pick up a roast. When I got there he was tying the meat with string. I noticed that his technique was very similar to my surgeon's suture tying, only he used his fingers and heavy white string. I asked him for some of the string and told him why I wanted it. He gave me a whole ball of it, asking only to be credited in the book. I'm not sure we did that, but I will give him credit here: Pergola's Meat Market on 7th Avenue in Brooklyn is, sadly, no longer in operation. I took the butcher's string home and began tying knots. Under the microscope it was easy to see what these knots looked like, no matter how many "throws" I made. Dr. Troutman thought I was a genius.

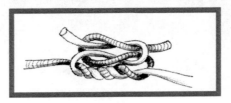

41

THE VITREOUS HUMOR

The posterior chamber is filled the vitreous humor. Unlike the aqueous humor, it is a gel, rather than a liquid. This gel has remarkable properties. It can be sifted through gauze and it comes out intact. It looks perfectly clear, but is made up of fibrils. It has no limiting membrane, but is simply more dense at its outside edges. It does not replenish itself. Once the vitreous humor is removed, the cavity created in the back of the eye fills with aqueous humor. The vitreous humor is attached at several places, the most adherent being just beneath the ora serrata. In youth it is attached to the base of the lens and around the macula, but in each of these places it releases with age. There is a canal that runs from the disc up to the central portion of the lens that, in the developing fetus, contains an artery called the hyloid artery. It serves no purpose once the baby is formed and the canal that remains is called the hyloid canal. The hyloid artery supplies the tiny vessels on the cornea in the developing fetus—the very ones I was asked by Dr. Fink to illustrate on the eyes of the little premature baby at the beginning of my career.

My Old Friend

Some patients cannot tolerate a contact lens and their vision problems are such that their glasses would be so thick that they would weigh much too heavily on the nose. Dr. Troutman developed a solution for these people. The donor cornea was frozen and refracted (shaped) to the specifications of the patient. Then a slit was cut in the recipient cornea, creating a pocket into which the donor cornea was slipped, like the filling in a sandwich. The procedure was so complex that Dr. Troutman recorded instructions on tape to be played as the surgeon operated, describing one step at a time. When I heard the name of the first patient on whom this surgery was to be tried, I was sure that I recognized it. He had been the photographer at my first wedding and a good friend of the family, but we had lost track of him. In fact, he had gone to a nursing home because he was going blind. He was also dying of cancer, but he volunteered for this surgery when he learned about it, as his eye condition was perfect for the procedure. I asked Dr. Troutman if I could visit this dear man after the surgery, and he said yes if the man could promise not to cry! Crying might undo all the doctor's careful work. I also was asked to wait for two days after surgery to give him a chance to start healing. Two days later I came back to the hospital. My dear old friend had been told I wished to visit him and he had agreed happily, promising not to cry. Of course I had to promise the same thing. Not fair if I cried and he couldn't. Emotions in check, I went into his hospital room. The lights were low and this tiny figure was sitting up in the bed. It had been at least 15 years since I had seen him. He told me he was seeing for the first time in five years, and what a blessing it was. He knew he had only a short time to live, but was grateful that those last weeks would be seeing ones, making his life ever so much easier and more satisfactory. We sat and held hands for a long while. I did not tell him the marriage he had photographed at its happy beginnings was in trouble. I promised to bring greetings to my husband and his family. I described our adorable children and the work I was now doing.

He died just three weeks later, but by volunteering to have the surgery he helped to show that it was a viable treatment for cases like his.

Corneal Graft part 7

Dr. Troutman now fixed the donor button in place with six evenly spaced interrupted sutures. Since the graft and site were round, it was read as a clock face with twelve o'clock at the top of the eye, that part nearest the surgeon. The first suture was placed at the six o'clock position, the second at twelve o'clock, the third at ten o'clock, the fourth at four o'clock, the fifth at two o'clock and the sixth at eight o'clock. This pattern of placement helped keep the donor button as evenly sutured at possible, like basting stitches that would be removed at the end of the finer suturing to come.

Interns and residents who are specializing in Ophthalmology and are learning how to do a corneal graft need a great deal of practice before they ever operate on a patient. Donated eyes that not good enough to use for a real graft are used for learning purposes. There are hardly enough of them to supply all the Fellows needing to practice surgery, so pig and cat eyes are used as well. A life-size mask is constructed with rubbery eyelids that are held open by a wire speculum, just as in real surgery. The practice eye is firmly attached to something like a hollowed out piece of cork that places the globe exactly behind the lids. A mask is used so that the learning surgeon can get used to working with the facial contours. A nose, especially a big one, can hamper the movement of the hands, and placing the sutures takes practice. Even when a Fellow has become adept in the laboratory, the first real surgery is still a momentous occasion. I remember one Fellow who took twenty minutes to make that first stitch. Dr. Troutman never hurried him, was there in case of need, encouraging every step of the way. This was probably the most impressive thing I watched in all my years of observing in the operating room—the incredible patience as the gift of this surgery was passed from the expert to the novice. I watched surgery performed by Dr. Troutman and his Fellows for over six years, once or twice a week. I never saw an error made; the precautions and training were that thorough and careful. This was not the place for anger, or impatience, or coffee for breakfast.

There are several suturing patterns used to sew in a graft and all of them are continuous sutures. The suturing begins at six o'clock and anywhere from 18 to 25 stitches are taken. There is one beautiful pattern created when a continuous suture is done in each direction. [Illustration 9.] This is used when the surgeon wants a particularly tight seal. The final knot (or knots) is buried in the recipient tissue so that nothing will irritate the inner lining of the lid or the donor tissue.

When suturing was finished, Dr. Troutman evened the individual bights by gently tugging on the sutures with a special forceps so that no part was tighter than any other. The object was to have the curvatures of the cornea the same in all directions. A device called a keratometer was mounted on the objective of the microscope. It had six or eight lights in a ring facing the cornea, which was reflected in the cornea. If the lights formed a perfect circle in the reflection then

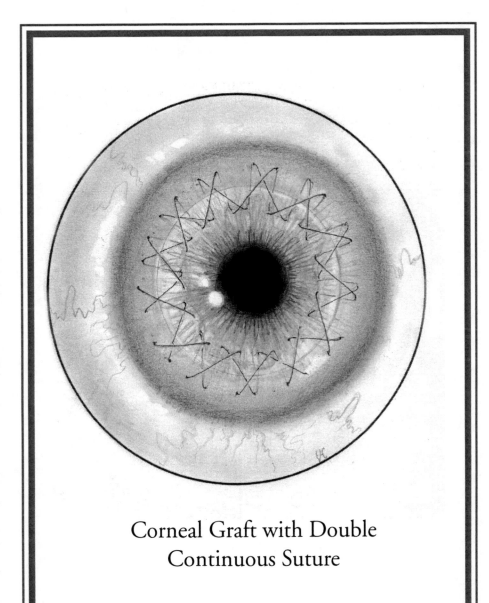

Corneal Graft with Double
Continuous Suture

Illustration 9

the surgeon knew he had an evenly sutured graft. If the reflection was an oval pattern, then the sutures were adjusted until a perfect circle could be seen.

Suddenly the surgery was over. The wire speculum was removed and a gauze patch taped gently over the eye. Then a metal shield with little holes in it, like a miniature colander, was taped over the eye, with the edges resting on the orbital rim to protect the remarkable surgery that had just been performed.

I have heard sad stories about brilliant surgeries that are successfully performed but then the patient fails to return for check-ups, or has an accident while drinking, undoing all that work.

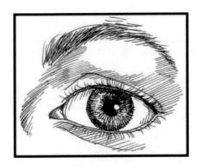

Chapter IV

External Structures

THE BONY ORBIT

*T*he two orbits are roughly cone-shaped; if you drew a line through the middle of each from the centers of the opening in front to the apexes in the rear and continued those lines backwards they would soon come to a point. The orbit is made up of seven different bones. They are the orbital plates of the sphenoid, ethmoid, and palatine bones; the maxilla; the frontal bone; the lacrimal bone, and the zygoma. I find it interesting that the dominant shape of the orbit has nothing to do with the shapes of the smaller pieces that make it up. They fit together like the pieces of a three dimensional jigsaw puzzle.

The vault formed by the frontal bone makes up the roof and nsasal side of the orbit. Just below it is the ethmoid bone and below that is the orbital plate of the maxilla. In front of them is the lacrimal bone and fossa, where the lacrimal sac resides. Just behind and between them you can see a tip of the palatine bone, which makes up a tiny portion of the floor of the orbit. The rest of the floor is made up of the orbital portion of the maxillary bone. The lateral wall is made up of the orbital plate of the great wing of the sphenoid bone behind, with the orbital portion of the zygomatic bone in front of it. At the very tip of the cone, above and just behind the vault of the frontal bone, is the lesser wing of the sphenoid bone.

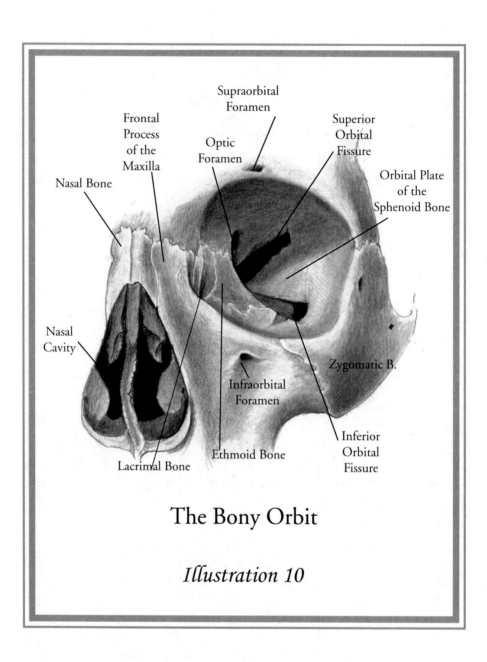

The Bony Orbit

Illustration 10

These bones are joined together at lines called sutures. Like the stitches that share their name, these sutures lock together, little fingers of bone meshing with opposing fingers of bone to create a solid joining.

There are holes and fissures in these bones which allow the vessels and nerves to enter the orbit. Right at the apex we see a round hole called the optic foramen, where the optic nerve exits from the back of the eye. This is the nerve that carries the information from the retina to the brain and back. There is another hole in the form of a V with the opening facing the lateral side of the orbit. The upper part is called the superior orbital fissure; the lower is called the inferior orbital fissure. There are two more small holes in the orbit along the suture line between the ethmoid and the frontal bones where nerves and vessels enter: the anterior and posterior ethmoidal foramina. A foramen means a small hole. Foramina is plural, from the Latin. [Illustration 10.]

The roof, the ethmoidal plate, and the maxillary orbital plates are very thin, especially the maxillary and ethmoid bones. A blow to the eye can cause these bones to break. The ethmoidal plate is so thin that it is translucent and you can faintly see the structures behind it. They are sinuses. [Illustration 11.]

GETTING ORGANIZED THE HARD WAY

I was hired by doctors Byron Smith and Dr. Frank Nesi to illustrate a two-volume text on Ophthalmic Plastic and Reconstructive Surgery. There were to be over 1500 illustrations with 57 contributing authors. Letters were sent out to all the participating doctors, giving them their assignments and introducing them to me as the medical illustrator with whom they would be working. Soon I was getting phone calls and the amount of information coming in was staggering. Before I even began to do the illustrations I had an accident. I was walking along 7th Avenue in Park Slope, Brooklyn where I lived, when I tripped and fell, hitting my head and knocking myself out. I came to as I was being loaded into an ambulance. From there I was taken to our local hospital's emergency room. During that short ride they peppered me questions

Getting Organized the Hard Way, continued

What was my name? I answered that everyone knew my name. How old was I? A lady doesn't tell her age. Who was president? Eisenhower came to mind. What was I doing on 7th Avenue? I hadn't a clue. I said, "Walking." A half-hour later my memory was beginning to return. At least I knew my name. My son was called and he came over to the hospital to take me home. They told me that I had a concussion and that I should not work for a week—to just take it easy. There was no question of working. I couldn't even if I wanted to. Instead, I used the time to get organized. When I was doing Troutman's second book I had had built a wonderful chest, about six feet in height, three feet wide and two-and-a- half feet deep with 20 open-faced drawers that slid in and out. I cleaned it out and labeled each drawer with the names of two or three authors. The drawers would hold the information coming in, the preliminary sketches, and the drawings as I finished them. Then I bought a good size cork board and pinned in one column the names of all the authors, a column for information coming in, a column for sketches done, a column for corrections done, and a column for finished art. This simple organization made keeping track of all the information manageable and was the system I used in all other big projects for the rest of my career.

Radial Keratometry Part 1

Eye surgery for centuries has depended on the surgeon's extraordinary manual skills. Now that the microscope has been introduced to ophthalmic surgery, the steadiness and accuracy of the hands have become even more important. Let's look at the surgery known as radial keratometry. This is surgery that makes little radial slices in the cornea which, when healed, change the shape of the cornea. Myopia or nearsightedness is corrected. These incisions are made by hand and require incredible steadiness and accuracy of pressure. The healing incisions flatten the cornea, correcting near- sightedness.

This is a much simpler procedure than a corneal graft. If all goes well, there is no penetration of the cornea; just neat little slits that stop, in depth, just short of Descemet's membrane and end at the limbus. The surgery can be done in a doctor's office if it is properly equipped with a small operating room and trained staff. The patient is given a topical anesthesia—a few drops on the cornea— which spreads to a little beyond the cornea. During the procedure, the eye must be stabilized; it is grasped with a special forceps at the scleral side of the limbus to keep the eye still.

HEADS IN WISCONSIN

The first chapter of the Smith/Nesi text was on anatomy. Instead of getting the material mailed to me, I was to go to Madison, Wisconsin, and work for ten days with Dr. Brad Lemke—dissecting heads.

I arrived on a beautiful summer day. After settling into my hotel room I went directly to Dr. Lemke's laboratory, a bright and airy room with tall windows that looked out over the campus. Dr. Lemke greeted me warmly, then showed me two huge jars filled with about 10 heads each. I looked out the window. I could see students riding their bicycles, some with tennis racquets strapped to the back, or swimming gear wadded in cases. Dr. Lemke made a ghoulish face and cackled, "Wouldn't they be surprised to know what we are doing up here. Heh heh heh."

Soon we were at work and we continued till dusk. The reason for so many heads is that there are always little differences in anatomy, especially the patterns of veins and arteries. We wanted to establish a norm by comparing as many as possible.

The next day we started our work early in the morning dissecting the meat off the bones to reveal the vessels and nerves of the first head. We broke for lunch. In the cafeteria I ordered a chicken salad sandwich. Dr. Lemke looked at the chicken meat and then at me, saying, "You're a better man than I am, Virginia," and he ordered a bowl of tomato soup.

THE SINUSES

Solid bone is heavy. If your skull were solid bone you would have trouble holding your head up. The skull is full of sinuses, which are cavities in the bones that surround the eye and drain into the nasal cavity. They are in so close to the orbit that trouble in one of them can affect the orbit. The reason you have them, troublesome as they can be, is that they decrease the density or weight of your skull.

The biggest sinus in the skull is the maxillary sinus, or antrum, in the maxilla. The ceiling of the antrum is the floor of the orbit. The bone separating them is quite thin and is one of the places where breakage is a danger to the integrity of the orbit and the eye. The floor of the antrum lies just above the roots of the molars and premolars. All of the sinuses are lined with mucous membrane and when irritated or infected produce mucous. If one of the sinuses is not able to drain easily, it causes pain and discomfort. That is why your teeth hurt if you have a sinus infection in the antrum.

Above the ceiling of the orbit is the frontal sinus, in the frontal bone. The frontal bone spans the forehead, creating the roofs of both orbits. The sinuses above the orbits are separated by a structure called the septum. There is great variety in their size. Drainage from these sinuses is through the infundibulum, a canal into the nasal cavity. Gravity is of help here, but problems can arise if the infundibulum becomes narrowed or clogged by infection. Also, the canal passes close to the drainage opening of the ethmoidal sinuses, and infection from one can spread easily to the others.

The ethmoidal plate forming the nasal wall of the orbit is paper-thin. You can see the septi—the walls of the bubble-like ethmoidal sinuses—behind that exterior surface of the bone. Because there are so many little compartments, not just one open space, there are three separate areas of drainage into the nasal cavity from these sinuses.

Behind the ethmoid bones are the sphenoids, the bodies of which are made up of the sphenoidal sinuses, just below the optic nerve. [Illustration 11.]

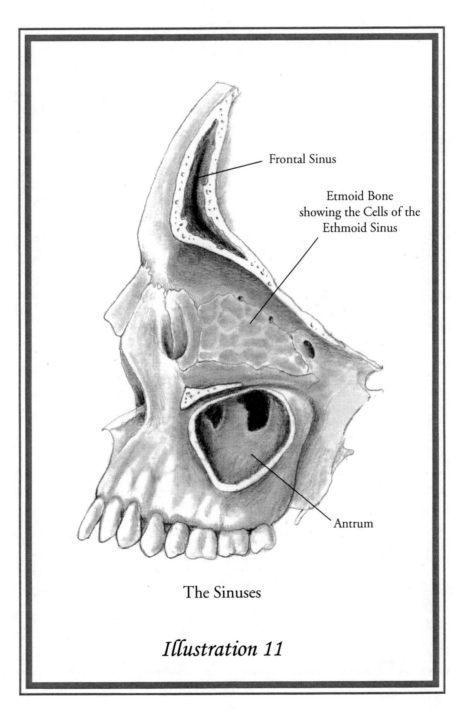

Frontal Sinus

Etmoid Bone
showing the Cells of the
Ethmoid Sinus

Antrum

The Sinuses

Illustration 11

MULTIBLE SCLEROSIS

One morning I woke to find I had trouble walking. Before then I had noticed my balance was getting bad—I had several falls, and I was losing my ability to ice skate—but that morning I found it hard to walk from one side of the room to the other. Stairs were an even greater challenge. I went to New York University's Department of Neurology where, after much testing, I was told I probably had Multiple Sclerosis (MS). I was devastated. I was crazy. I didn't know how to accept this news. I was a physically active person who loved to dance, to hike, to skate, to build things, to do. I was the one who painted our house. It all was wiped out in a day. Suddenly I needed a cane to walk, a wheelchair to get around any distance, and picking up anything that weighed more than ten pounds was out of the question.

I was in the middle of the text on Ocular Plastic and Reconstructive Surgery. I tried to work but could not concentrate. I wanted to find other doctors who would give me better news or more helpful information. I called Dr. Smith and Dr. Nesi as well as Eugenia Klein at Mosby to tell them of the diagnosis and how hard I was finding it to work. Then I was frightened that I had made a big mistake by revealing my situation.

I hadn't. They all said not to worry, I should take what time I needed to pursue help. They would wait for me, as they wanted me to do the drawings. They told me no one could do them better and they knew I would be able to do them in time. The relief I felt was enormous. I did go see other doctors, but I also began working again on the book. In fact, I was able to finish it by the original deadline

I learned that Eugenia had polio when a young woman. Years later she experienced post-polio syndrome, a condition in which some polio symptoms return years later. The next time we met at a conference, we were both in wheelchairs.

The surgery begins with the establishment of the optical center, of the cornea directly over the pupil. The center is lightly marked with a dull needle, which makes a dent, not a puncture. Then the whole "optical zone" is marked with an instrument that looks like a ring with cross-hairs and a handle. When the cross-hairs show that the instrument is properly centered, it is lowered onto the cornea and turned, leaving a circular mark 3 to 4 mm in diameter on the surface of the cornea. The edge of the ring is dull, so it doesn't damage the cornea but leaves a groove in the epithelium. That mark will disappear later. This mark limits the length of the incisions. If the incisions are made too close to the optical zone, the patient will experience a disturbing glare. For this reason, when the incisions are made they go from the marked ring outward.

Three very critical points make for the success of this surgery. First is the steadiness and accuracy of the surgeon. Second is the accuracy of the measurements—of the center of the visual part of the cornea and the depth of the cornea; the length of the blade must be tailored to the cornea's depth. Last, the surgeon must be sure that the knife blade is absolutely clean and unmarred. This surgery was originally done with a razor knife blade. Now the knife of choice is the diamond knife. The cutting surface is easily damaged if not properly cleaned. If there is a minute bit of old tissue still on the blade it will just harden in the autoclave (the sterilizing machine). It is very easy to chip this blade, particularly the entering point. Before any cutting is done, the knife must be carefully examined to be sure that nothing will impede its perfect path through the cornea. While the knife is handheld, the handle that clasps the blade is made with a guard to protect the knife and insure that it will only enter to the desired depth. Usually eight incisions are made, equally spaced, radiating from the centrally marked circle. The closer they are to the center of the eye, the more they flatten the cornea.

A protective bandage is put over the eye and a therapeutic contact lens is put on the cornea, eliminating most of the pain and hastening recovery. The patient can see fairly well right after surgery.

THE EYELIDS

The eye is the one exposed organ of the body, if you don't count the skin. It needs constant care and protection, which is provided automatically by the eyelids. [Illustration 12.]

The lid movement is made possible by three muscles: a circular one around the eye, and two others that come from deep in the orbit to attach to the tarsus—the structure that stiffens each lid and is found in the area just behind the lashes.

The first muscle is called the orbicularis oculi. The fibers of this muscle attach to a tendon on the nasal side of the lid, and on the lateral or outer side they form what is called a raphé, where the upper fibers mesh with those coming from below. The orbicularis of the upper lid is divided into two portions: the orbital portion, and the outermost rings of fibers, called the palpebral portion. Palpebra is Latin for eyelids. The entire muscle is a sphincter or circular muscle. It is the one we use when we close our eyes. The palpebral part closes them, controlling the blinking action; the orbital portion is what we use when we close our eyes tightly, or squint.

The second lid muscle is called the levator (palpebra superioris). Its origin of attachment is the roof of the orbit deep inside the cavity, and from the orbital surface of the lesser wing of the sphenoid bone. It courses forward over the eye, lying right on top of the superior rectus muscle. As it reaches the front of the orbit, it becomes tendinous and fans out in a thin fibrous sheath called an aponeurosis. It covers the entire front of the eye when the lids are closed. The attachments of insertion are to the front of the tarsus, with fibers that peel off the lower portion of the aponeurosis, filtering through the muscle fiber bundles of the orbicularis, to attach to the underside of the skin. It opens the eye by lifting the lid, acting to counter the action of the orbicularis. The attachment to the skin creates the lid crease.

Running just under the aponeurosis and attached at its origin to the underside of the levator is a small flat muscle that inserts along the outer border of the tarsus, called Müller's Muscle. It too assists in lifting the upper lid. There is a similar muscle in the lower lid, even smaller and less effective, that originates from the fibers of the inferior rectus muscle and attaches to the outer border of the tarsus of the lower lid. I have heard surgeons debating whether there is, in

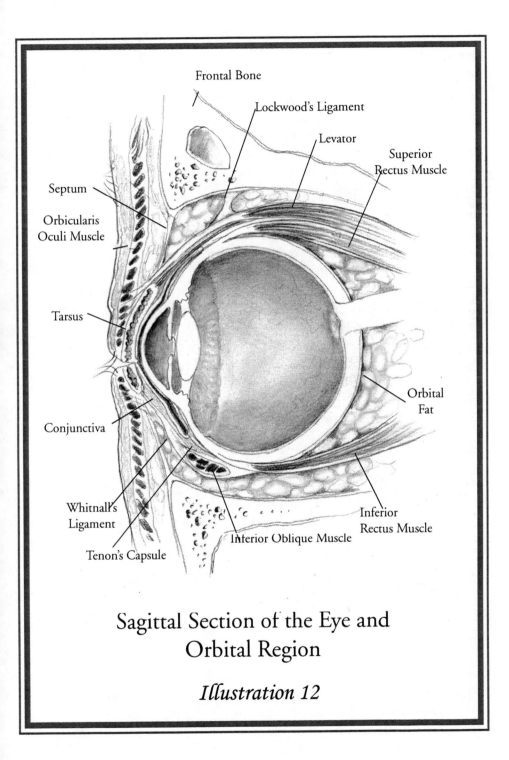

Sagittal Section of the Eye and Orbital Region

Illustration 12

fact, a Müller's Muscle in the lower lid. In some it is more apparent than in others.

Both the upper and lower lids have the stiffening fibrous structures called tarsi (singular: tarsus). If you take a match stick or cotton swab you can fold the upper lid over it, a rather ghastly looking thing to do but as kids we loved doing it, hoping to terrify our parents. The underside of the tarsus is lined with the conjunctiva, which is very red and vascularized—full of arteries and veins.

The tarsus of the upper lid is taller than that of the lower lid, being almost twice the size from margin to border. Embedded in the tarsi are glands that look like strings of beads with the strings all lying parallel to each other. They are called Meibomian glands and have little openings on the lid margins that secrete sebum. With every blink a slightly oily surface is laid down over the moisture of the tears already spread over the cornea, to slow their evaporation. It is important that the cornea be kept moist but not too moist, just enough so that it retains its proper thickness and doesn't dehydrate. The oily sebum helps to prevent the tears from spilling out and insures an airtight seal when the eyes are closed. The toughness of the tarsi and their curvature, which matches the curvature of the cornea, help to protect the eye.

Attached to the tarsus in the lower lid and the tarsus in the upper lid is a thin tissue called the orbital septum, which separates the contents of the orbit from the muscle and skin of the lids. The septum attaches at the orbital rim and to the levator just above the tarsus in the upper lid. In the lower lid it attaches to the inferior border of the tarsus. The septum holds in place the fat that fills the orbit. That fat protects the eye. Every organ has its protective fat. Problems can arise in the orbit, as it is a very limited space with only one direction for things to go—forward. That means baggy eyelids, and even eyes that bulge out if things get too packed in there.

The ends of the tarsi become tendinous bands. On the lateral side, these bands, called the lateral canthal tendons, join and attach to the orbital rim. On the side near the nose they join at the anterior lacrimal crest and go on to attach to the frontal process of the maxilla, the bone found just at the side of the nose. These bands hold the lids in place. If either side becomes stretched or lax, there

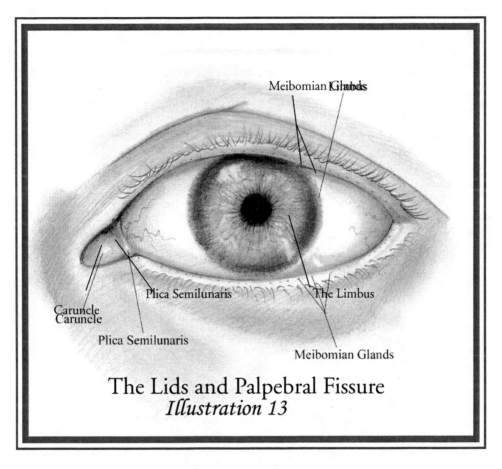

Meibomian Glands

Plica Semilunaris

The Limbus

Caruncle

Plica Semilunaris

Meibomian Glands

The Lids and Palpebral Fissure
Illustration 13

is trouble keeping the lids closed properly.

The opening between the lids is called the palpebral fissure through which you see the eye when it is open. [Illustration 13.] That opened fissure is a fusiform or football-like shape. The ends are called the canthi (singular: canthus). There's not much going on at the lateral canthus, but the medial canthus has a lot going on and it doesn't come neatly to a point. At the very angle of the medial canthus is a pink little mound called the caruncle, and next to it is a fold of pink tissue called the plica semilunaris. The caruncle has some lacrimal (tear) and sebaceous glands and the plica is a fold of conjunctiva-like tissue that opens and closes as the eye turns back and forth. Plicare means "to fold" in Latin. It is the caruncle that produces the fluid that dries to make the "sand" in your eyes.

The time had come for me to become a member of the Association of Medical Illustrators. Qualifying for membership was not easy. The candidates had to be sponsored and were required to submit examples of art work—eight or 10 illustrations.

I knew I had two strikes against me. First, I left college in the middle of my junior year to attend The Boston Museum School of Fine Arts; I had no formal degree. Second, I would be competing with graduates of recognized schools of medical illustration with Masters degrees. To apply at all, a candidate had to be sponsored by three people within the AMI and one person from outside the organization. My sponsors were a former president of the organization and two members in good standing suggested by him. My outside sponsor was Dr. Troutman who by then, because of our books, was the leading corneal surgeon in the country. I thought I was a shoo-in.

The drawings were to be mailed to the membership chairman who would bring them to the meeting. I remember thinking I would not mat the drawings so that they would be easier for her to carry. Little did I know. I went to the meeting feeling shy but confident. I met fellow medical illustrators and attended courses to improve my skills. On the last day, in front of the whole membership, the new members were named and welcomed into the fold. I was not among them. I was devastated. I went stumbling back to my room in tears. There was a knock on my door. The membership chairman had come to tell me that she felt terrible about what had happened. All the graduate students of the schools of medical illustration had been instructed to mat their submissions. I, of course, never got those instructions.

She urged me to take a junior membership for the next year and re-apply the following year. She also suggested that I get as sponsors those people who had voted me down this year. What a good idea! I dried my eyes and thanked her. I took her advice. The following year my portfolio was impeccable and I was accepted.

I later learned that Frank Netter, the most famous medical illustrator in the country, had been turned down for membership when he first applied because he felt he didn't need to supply a portfolio. Later, wiser minds within the organization invited him to join.

Strabismus

Strabismus is a misalignment of the eyes. The condition we are most familiar with is cross-eyes, where both of the eyes look inward. But there are many other configurations.

Surgery can correct many of these problems. The surgery is usually done on one of the rectus muscles, those muscles attached to the eye in the north, south, east, and west positions. One muscle can be shortened, or the opposing muscle can be lengthened. A careful evaluation is done to decide just how to approach the problem and which method will bring the desired result. To shorten a muscle, either a pleat or tuck can be made in it. To lengthen a muscle, cuts can be made in it so that it will stretch out. The muscle attachment to the globe can also be changed by cutting it off from its original attachment and suturing it either farther forward or farther back, depending on what is needed.

When a child has a strabismus problem and the eyes are very different in orientation, only one eye is used at a time, so the child doesn't have stereoscopic vision. If both eyes are used, the child sees double. It is important to correct this problem as soon as possible or the brain loses the capacity for depth perception.

When I started my first book with Dr. Troutman, I was married and not thinking of my work as my business. By the time I was in the middle of our second book, I was thinking of divorce and realizing that I had to change my approach to what I was doing. I had to learn how to run a business. I also decided that I had to know as much as I could about the eye. One of the things that may have contributed to the end of my marriage, that little fillip that tips the load, was the evening when I handed my husband his martini with a glass eye in the bottom staring back at him instead of an olive. He was lucky—I had been considering a real one.

I often brought donor eyes home from the eye bank where they knew I was working with Dr. Troutman and were cooperative. When there was a donated eye that couldn't be used for surgery, and all the Fellows had as many as they needed for their practice sessions, they would let me take one or two home. They gave them to me in a paper packet similar to a Chinese food take-out container. I would mark the container so that no one would make a mistake: "IF YOU WANT TO THROW UP LOOK INSIDE." My family was not as tough as I had become. I learned to dissect the eye under the microscope, using the instruments Dr. Troutman had given me. Or I would freeze eyes and slice them to see how a sagittal section would look.

One of the ways I set up my drawings was to put a glass eye on a ball of clay and then look at it under the microscope. A glass eye is not round, not even a half sphere. Dr. Troutman had arranged for me to have the same kind of microscope with which the Fellows trained. In that way I could be sure the proportions were right. Instruments that looked tiny as they lay in their case looked enormous under the microscope.

Having one's own surgical microscope had other advantages. In the summer when we moved to the country in upstate New York, we would look at bees or caterpillars, mosquitoes or beetles—whatever tiny fauna we found expired around our place. Butterfly wings under the microscope are almost as beautiful as the human iris.

FAINTING

The one time I fainted in surgery was after I had been observing Dr. Troutman for over a year. I'd seen corneal grafts, cataract surgery, glaucoma surgery, trauma surgery (a piece of a bullet shell was embedded in a man's eye, just behind the iris and there had been much trouble finding it. They did, but that is another story). I thought I was pretty hot stuff, and ready for anything. I came into the operating room this particular morning and the whole setup was different. The ceiling-mounted microscope was still "in bed" and Dr. Troutman was wearing loupes. The instruments on the instrument tray looked unfamiliar—too big, as they weren't microsurgical instruments. Dr. Troutman explained that he had begun his training as a plastic surgeo and had switched to ophthalmic surgery later, looking for a greater challenge I suppose. The patient was a doctor friend who wanted him, Troutman, to do a blepharoplasty for him. Bleph, as it is called for short, is surgery to remove the bags under and over the eyes and to remove the redundant skin that forms as we grow older. For starters, with the first incision that went in the upper lid, there was—blood! Corneal surgery has very little of the stuff, but when you cut into skin, there is a lot. A cautery was used to stanch the flow, zap zap, with little puffs of smoke and a smell of burning flesh. A sort of lozenge shape of tissue was removed from the upper lid, the septum was pierced, and all of sudden there was a glob of yellow fat came popping out. I was gone. I awoke on a gurney in the recovery room with a nurse asking me if I'd had breakfast. Of course I'd had breakfast. It was that blood and that fat! I tested my equilibrium by sitting up. That worked. I stood up. That worked. I found my way to the very operating room where I had collapsed about 10 minutes before. When I went in Dr. Troutman slightly raised his head and said, "Clean up the blood, here comes Virginia."

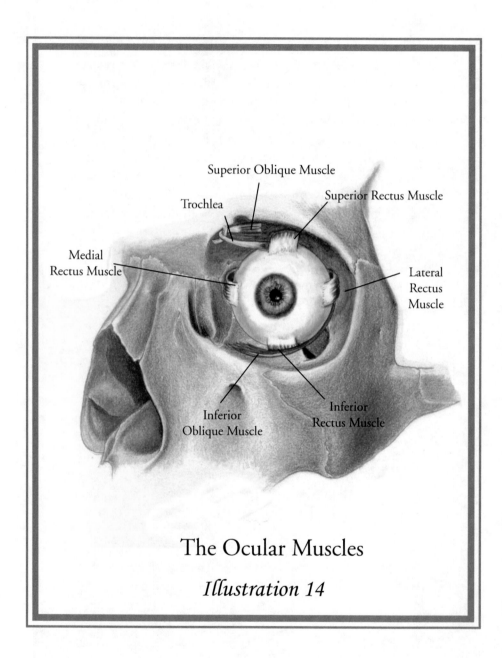

The Ocular Muscles

Illustration 14

THE OCULAR MUSCLES

There are six muscles that attach to the globe, inserted in the sclera. Four of them are simply front-to-back muscles. These are located at north, south, east, and west and are called the superior, inferior, lateral, and medial rectus muscles. These muscles course back to attach to a circular tendon, called the annulus of Zinn, found at the apex of the orbit anchored to the sphenoid bone. The muscles are flat and rectangular. More subtle movement is controlled by two other muscles, the inferior and superior oblique muscles. The inferior oblique muscle arises, or begins, on the orbital plate of the maxilla just behind the lacrimal duct. It goes under the globe at an oblique angle to insert on the globe just behind the vertical meridian and below the horizontal one. Its opposite is the superior rectus muscle, which is a truly fascinating muscle because it works like a pulley, not in a direct fashion as almost all other muscles do. It originates from the annulus of Zinn back at the apex of the orbit, covering the origin of the levator. It courses forward as a round muscle, then becomes a tendon, which goes through a loop attached to the medial wall of the orbit just behind the rim. After going through this loop, called the trochlea, it turns back to attach to the globe just under the superior rectus muscle in a fanned-out shape. [Illustration 14.]

The Animal Ophthalmologist

Just two weeks after I separated from my husband, I went to a conference of ophthalmology, called the Academy, given every year to bring the doctors together to take courses, attend lectures, and stroll through the enormous hall devoted to exhibitions of research, as well as the products manufactured for all aspects of ophthalmic surgery. Ophthalmologists gather from all over the world to attend the yearly Academies. This particular year it was in held Las Vegas. A few weeks before the conference I was contacted by an animal ophthalmologist to do some drawings for him, and we planned to meet at the academy where he would look at what I had done, going over them for corrections. We met at a coffee shop in the hotel. After we finished our business he asked me

The Animal Ophthalmologist, continueed

to go out for dinner, and then made a serious offer to meet me every Monday evening in New York City for the experience of my lifetime. My eyes got wide and my insides said "get out of here." I thanked him profusely for his kind offer but declined. Still he pressed his case with vivid descriptions of what I would enjoy. I excused myself as politely as I could and fled to my room. I saw that my life as a single woman had begun. When the drawings were finally finished and delivered, the animal ophthalmologist paid promptly with a little note saying he was sorry things hadn't worked out.

My children had begged me not to gamble while in Las Vegas. They were feeling very insecure in this new situation. At the airport, as I was leaving, I put two quarters in a slot and won a dollar on each, which I took home to them.

Cataract Surgery

A cataract is formed when the lens of the eye becomes opaque, obscuring vision. You may have seen dogs or cats with this condition. The pupil looks white or cloudy instead of black. Cataracts can affect vision even before they become noticeable, so they are among the things an ophthalmologist looks for during a routine eye exam.

Cataract surgery has been performed since ancient times. In ancient Rome an incision was made in the cornea with a rather crude knife and the offending lens was removed. The cornea was left to heal on its own. There was no anesthesia. Even in fairly modern times the surgery was harrowing. The patient had to lie still for days while the cornea healed, head held motionless. After that the person had to wear glasses with lenses so thick they looked like the bottoms of old fashioned soft drink bottles.

At the time I started watching cataract surgery, lens implants had been invented but were not as safe as the ones used today and therefore rarely used. In almost all cases, one eye was done at a time, letting the first eye heal before removing the cataract from the second eye. This meant that the patient had to spend some weeks, if not months, with each eye seeing differently. With the lens removed, objects appear much bigger. The difference would often cause the person to feel ill. Those early lens implant surgeries also required big incisions extending all the way from the "three o'clock" position to the "nine o'clock" position. The closure, no matter how carefully sutured, usually left an astigmatism—an irregularity in the cornea—that affected vision. The lens was removed with a spatula- like instrument especially designed for the task, or later with a cryoprobe that had a tip that could be chilled to below freezing so it would stick to the lens, enabling the probe to pull it out. This surgery was called intracapsular cataract extraction because the capsule that covers the lens was removed with the lens. Later it was felt that it was better to leave the capsule in place, still attached to the zonules. The capsule tissue is like clear plastic wrap, and it was easy enough to cut a hole allowing the lens to be removed while leaving the capsule behind. This was called extracapsular cataract extraction and is the most popular way of doing this surgery today. The remaining capsule separates the back from the front of the eye and provides a convenient "bag" in which to place the lens implant.

Early implants were designed to sit on the iris. Little plastic arms called haptics were embedded in the lens and stuck out on either side to hold the lens in place. These haptics were placed in the angle of the eye and often caused problems there, sometimes interfering with that drainage system—the trabecular meshwork—that is so important to maintaining the even pressure of the eye. Some implants had dramatic shapes. One was nicknamed "the pregnant seven" for its distinctive contours. Dr. CharlesKelman, who 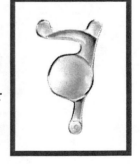 designed it, went on to invent another tool that revolutionized cataract surgery, but the pregnant seven was not a success.

Today cataract surgery is so quick and easy that it is often done as an out-patient procedure, requiring only local anesthesia. The lens is removed with a "phacoemulsifier," invented by Dr.Kelman. A very small incision is made, just large enough for the phacoemulsifier to fit though. The instrument is able to emulsify—or break up—the cataract into small pieces, which are then sucked out of the eye by the probe tip, leaving the clear capsule in place. Next the interocular lens is introduced in a collapsed form. Once placed behind the pupil, it opens up, with the new lens directly behind the pupil and the haptics reaching into the edges of the lens capsule.

Sometimes the normally clear lens capsule turns cloudy. This is called a secondary cataract. A laser is used to clear away the cloudy capsule in the area behind the pupil so no new surgery is needed.

The advantages of the IOL, the interocular lens implant, are many. The vision that is restored to the eye is the same, if not better, than what the person enjoyed before developing cataracts. While one eye is healing, the image appears the same size in both eyes, eliminating the earlier problem of nausea caused by the difference in vision between the treated and untreated eyes. Overall vision can often be improved. This is what happened to my cousin. He had been very near-sighted all of his life, wearing thick glasses, and nearly blind without them. After the surgery he needed glasses only for reading.

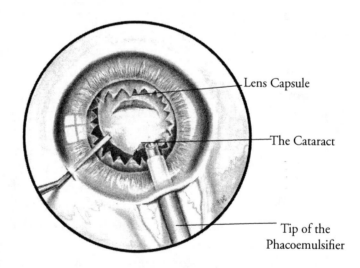

Lens Capsule

The Cataract

Tip of the
Phacoemulsifier

Illustration 15

Illustration 15 shows the phacoemulsifier probe tip (on the right) removing a piece of the cataract. The instrument on the left is used to steady the lens. The jagged edge shows where the lens capsule has been cut away, You can see how small the incision is and therefore how easily it can heal, sometimes without suturing. My illustration is taken from the *Atlas of Contemporary Ophthalmic Surgery,* by Henry Clayman.

MOON

Dr. Troutman and Dr.Kelman shared the same floor at
the Manhattan Eye and Ear Hospital, where there was a
whole wing devoted to the library and research. Dr. Troutman always took the staircase to the seventh floor, two
steps at a time. Dr.Kelman and I took the elevator, and
one day we shared it. He told me he had found a wonderful illustrator, a man who called himself "Moon" and who
was a genius with the airbrush. It seems Dr.Kelman had
found him in the 42nd Street and Broadway area doing
air brush drawings of lascivious nudes. Dr.Kelman was
doing a book on how to use the phacoemulsifier and hired
Moon to illustrate the book. He had installed Moon in his
own studio in the hospital annex in a room right next to
where all the cats to be used for experimental surgery were
kept. Dr.Kelman asked me if I would like to meet Moon.
I wouldn't have missed that opportunity for anything.
I was curious about how he was dealing with the howl-
ing cats after a life on 42nd Street. As I suspected, Moon
was going out of his mind. The moment Dr.Kellman left
us alone in Moon's little gray cubicle-studio, Moon began rolling his eyes heavenward, telling me the place was
driving him nuts. Dr.Kelman was paying him so well he
couldn't afford to quit, but he wasn't sure his sanity would
last the book.

Moon looked like a character from 42nd Street. He
had a black silk bandanna tied around his head, a seldom
washed ragged wool shirt and dungarees that were full of
holes long before it was fashionable. He had a wild look
in his eye and it wouldn't have surprised me if he kept
himself from going insane on some illicit drug. He could
wield an airbrush, however, and did a creditable job on
Dr.Kelman's book. But the moment that last drawing was
done, paycheck in hand, he was out of there.

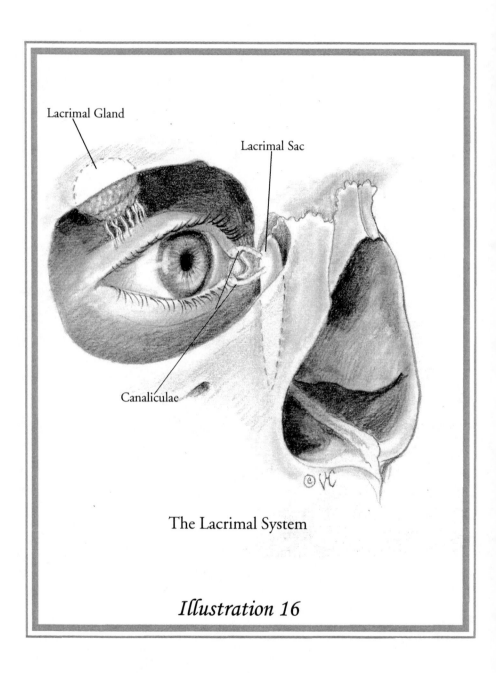

Lacrimal Gland

Lacrimal Sac

Canaliculae

The Lacrimal System

Illustration 16

THE LACRIMAL SYSTEM

The lacrimal system is made up of the glands that produce tears and the apparatus that clears them away.

The lacrimal gland is found above and lateral (to the outside) of each eye. It is bi-lobed; that is, it is in two parts. One part is above the levator and the other beneath it. They are connected by tiny ducts and the lower one has more little ducts that spill the tears into the eye. The gland is the size of a small nut, and is made up of many lobules in which the tears are made and then sent into their passageways. This is the gland that goes into action when we cry. It produces so much fluid that the drainage system cannot handle it all nor can the natural barriers created by the meibomian gland secretions in the tarsus [see section on lids, p. 56], so the tears spill over. In the conjunctiva, particularly the upper lid, there are also clusters of lacrimal gland cells that produce tears on a regular basis and that keep the front of the globe moist, along with the oily sebum produced by the meibomian glands. These tears do not spill over, but are drained off through minute holes called the puncti (singular: punctum) in both the upper and lower lids, located near the medial canthus. The puncti are openings at the end of the canaliculae (small tube-like canals) that feed into the lacrimal sac. When we were looking at the skull we saw the lacrimal bone, which joined with the frontal process of the maxilla creating the lacrimal fossa, or hole, in which the sac sits. The sac drains off the tears into the nasal cavity. Gravity is helpful here but so is the action of blinking. The orbicularis muscle fibers pass over the sac and with each blink provide a pumping action that draws the fluid in and pushes it out into the nasal cavity. Sometimes extra tears are produced from the cold, from eating, and from crying, and that runny nose includes tears, not just mucous. [Illustration 16.]

Tears are slightly salty. That is why water in your eyes isn't comfortable for them. A saline solution feels much better and that is what is used during corneal surgery—a fluid that mimics tears.

SUSPENSORY LIGAMENTS AND TENON'S CAPSULE

When you think about it, the eye is being turned by six different muscles, but in spite of all that tugging and releasing of muscles, the globe stays in the same place; it doesn't get pulled up or down, to the side or backwards, but rolls around in a stable position. Part of that is the exquisite relationship of the muscles themselves, but part is because the globe is suspended and held in place by ligaments that wrap around it like a hammock underneath— Lockwood's Ligament—and a band of tissue over the top— Whitnall's Ligament. Both ligaments are attached at either side, near or on the tendons that come off the lids at the canthi—the medial canthal and lateral canthal tendons, discussed earlier. A myriad of almost undetectable suspensory ligaments all around the eye aid in keeping the eye in place as it rolls around. The eye also is encased within Tenon's capsule, which rolls around with the globe, as it is attached to the globe just behind the limbus and over the recti muscles. The orbital fat plays a role in maintaining the position of the eye. The orbit is packed with it and the suspensory ligaments run through that fat, holding it in place as it holds the globe in place.

UNCOVERING A MURDER

One of the ways that I learned about the anatomy of the eye and its orbit was through participating in dissections. If you are faint of heart, you might want to skip this section, but then you'll miss a wonderful story.

For medical students, more emphasis is placed on the anatomy of the rest of the body, starting from the neck down. Only specialists concentrate on the head—those studying the brain for instance, plastic surgeons, and those who specialize in the area surrounding the eye. I was invited by Dr. Della Rocca to attend several dissections. He was an anatomist as well as a fine surgeon, and part of his commitment as a doctor was to pass on to his Fellows the knowledge that he had gained through dissection.

Obtaining cadaver material is not easy. People have to donate their bodies, or people whose bodies are not claimed are sometimes used for medical dissection and anatomical studies. The unclaimed bodies are not very pretty. They are usually people who have lived a homeless life for years and die of alcoholism and exposure. So right off, the sight of the specimen is off-putting. The head is severed from the body. We didn't need the rest of the body—it could be used by other medical students for their own purposes. We had three heads, in this case, and nine Fellows, including myself. Since heads are symmetrical for the most part, the heads were then cut in two, right through the nose, longitudinally. Three of us were assigned to a half a head. When we saw our half, we could see that there was a hemorrhage in the frontal lobe of the brain and we quickly agreed that we knew how the person had died, and went on about our business. I found I was so curious to actually see what I had for so long been drawing—studying from other people's drawings, studying from watching surgery, reading descriptions, or listening to what doctors explained to me—that I overcame any feelings of repulsion or faintness and was very aware of everything that was happening.

The room in which we worked lacked charm. It had kitchen-green walls and black tile floors. Long metal tables were where we worked, and steadying a half a head on a metal table was no mean feat. The heads were wet and slippery. The Fellow who was doing the dissection on our head became impatient with trying to prop up and steady our half a head so he asked me to grasp the hair and hold it firm. We were wearing rubber gloves, so there was protection. I did as I was told and then noticed a little hole in the scalp where the hair parted. I asked for a probe, and sure enough, it went right down to that place in the brain where we could see the hemorrhage. I had discovered a murder! A little inquiry revealed that our head was irrevocably separated from its body and no one knew where the body was, and this was someone found on the streets, unclaimed, many months before. No one would be interested in the murder of this poor soul. We found no bullet, so we surmised that the man had been struck with an ice pick or something similar.

I was impressed with how quickly my team was back at the task at hand, and we all learned a great deal about the structures surrounding the eye, much of which I have been describing.

THE VASCULAR AND NEURAL SUPPLY

The blood supply to the eye and surrounding tissues comes from the inner and outer carotid arteries. The vessels find their way into the orbit via the optic foramen, the hole in the back of the orbit where the optic nerve enters. They also enter through the superior and inferior orbital fissures. Other vessels find their way across the face and onto the lids.

The neural system for the ocular area is supplied by the various cranial nerves, of which there are many branches. They too find their way into the orbit through the orbital fissures, as well as traveling to the face where they become the facial nerve. There are two kinds of nerves: the motor nerves that cause muscles to move, and the sensory nerves that cause feeling and sight.

. Illustrations 17 and 18 were done for the anatomy chapter of Byron Smith's text: *Ocular Plastic and Reconstructive Surgery* discussed in my anecdote "Heads in Wisconsin."

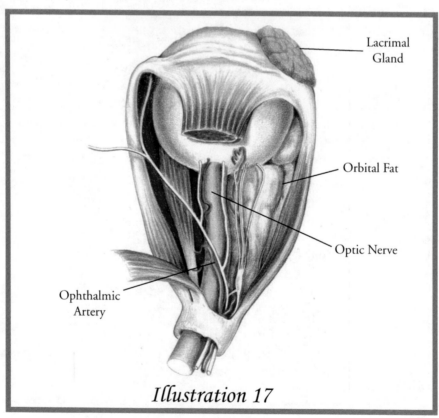

Lacrimal Gland

Orbital Fat

Optic Nerve

Ophthalmic Artery

Illustration 17

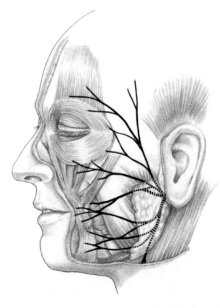

Facial Nerves

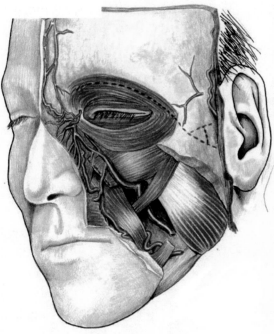

Facial Arteries
and Veins

Illustration 18

My mother used to say, "All good things come to an end." And so, at the right time, did my career. When I began medical illustrating, C.V. Mosby was an entity in itself, as was W.B. Saunders. They were devoted to medical publishing. Their editors could speak the language and understand what was being written about. They visited the operating rooms to observe surgery. It was a pleasure dealing with them.

Then these as well as other medical publishing houses were bought up by larger companies, which in turn were bought by larger ones. The new editors seemed concerned with bottom line only. One of them asked me to give them a bulk rate. I replied that I was not the Post Office. It stopped being fun and turned into grim business. Working with the doctors did not change, of course, but we were all growing older. Many of the doctors I worked with for so long were retiring. I didn't pursue finding new clients. I let it go. It was time for me to retire too. When I finished my last book, a text called *Ocular Plastic Surgery*, I just put down my pen and started painting. Now and then one of my former clients will ask me to do some drawings and I will do it happily. Doing this book has been like recalling what it used to be like. I find I am as hard a task master as any of the doctors I worked for and I have loved getting organized once again with a shelf in my chest devoted to the illustrations. I have loved revisiting that intriguing, fascinating landscape of the eye.

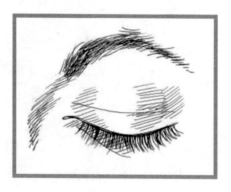